T0292385

Atlas *of* SEXUAL VIOLENCE

Atlas *of*
SEXUAL
VIOLENCE

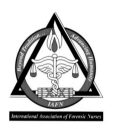

International Association
of Forensic Nurses

Tara Henry, **MSN, FNP-C, SANE-A, SANE-P**
Volume Editor

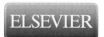

3251 Riverport Lane
St. Louis, Missouri 63043

ATLAS OF SEXUAL VIOLENCE   ISBN: 978-1-4377-2783-8

Notices

Knowledge and best practice in this field are constantly changing. As new research and experience broaden our understanding, changes in research methods, professional practices, or medical treatment may become necessary.

Practitioners and researchers must always rely on their own experience and knowledge in evaluating and using any information, methods, compounds, or experiments described herein. In using such information or methods they should be mindful of their own safety and the safety of others, including parties for whom they have a professional responsibility.

With respect to any drug or pharmaceutical products identified, readers are advised to check the most current information provided (i) on procedures featured or (ii) by the manufacturer of each product to be administered, to verify the recommended dose or formula, the method and duration of administration, and contraindications. It is the responsibility of practitioners, relying on their own experience and knowledge of their patients, to make diagnoses, to determine dosages and the best treatment for each individual patient, and to take all appropriate safety precautions.

To the fullest extent of the law, neither the Publisher nor the authors, contributors, or editors, assume any liability for any injury and/or damage to persons or property as a matter of products liability, negligence or otherwise, or from any use or operation of any methods, products, instructions, or ideas contained in the material herein.

Library of Congress Cataloging-in-Publication Data
Atlas of sexual violence / Tara Henry.
       p. cm.
   Includes bibliographical references and index.
   ISBN 978-1-4377-2783-8 (alk. paper)
   1. Sexual abuse victims--Wounds and injuries. 2. Sexual abuse victims--Physiology. 3. Rape victims--Medical examinations. 4. Generative organs--Wounds and injuries. I. Henry, Tara.
   RC560.S44A85 2012

616.85'83--dc23

                                                                    2011052989

Acquisitions Editor: Sandra Clark
Developmental Editor: Charlene Ketchum
Publishing Services Manager: Jeff Patterson
Senior Project Manager: Anne Konopka
Design Direction: Ashley Eberts

Printed in the United States of America

Last digit is the print number: 9   8   7   6   5   4   3   2   1

CONTRIBUTORS

Susan Chasson, MSN, JD, SANE-A
Family Nurse Practitioner
Merrill Gappmayer Family Medicine Center
and
Lecturer
College of Nursing
Brigham Young University
Provo, Utah

Kim Day, RN, FNE, SANE-A, SANE-P
SAFE Technical Assistance Coordinator
International Association of Forensic Nurses
Arnold, Maryland

Renae Diegel, RN, BBL, CEN, CFN, CMI-III, D-ABMDI, SANE-A, CFC, DABFN, DABFE
Medical Examiner Investigator
Macomb County Medical Examiner's Office
Mt. Clemens, Michigan
and
Forensic Nurse Examiner/Educator
Turning Points Forensic Nurse Examiner Program
Clinton Township, Michigan

Christine Dunnuck, RN, MSN, FNP-BC, SANE-A
Coordinator, Nurse Examiner Program
YWCA West Central Michigan
Grand Rapids, Michigan

Tara Henry, MSN, FNP-C, SANE-A, SANE-P
Forensic Nurse Services
Anchorage, Alaska

Jeffrey Jones, MD, FACEP
Professor, Division of Emergency Medicine
MSU College of Human Medicine
Grand Rapids, Michigan

Jenifer Markowitz, ND, RN, WHNP-BC, DF-IAFN
Medical Advisor
Aequitas: The Prosecutor's Resource on
Violence Against Women
Washington, DC

Linda Rossman, RN, MSN, WHNP-BC, PNP-BC, SANE-A, SANE-P
Manager: Nurse Examiner Program
YWCA West Central Michigan
Grand Rapids, Michigan

Daniel J. Spitz, MD
Chief Medical Examiner
Macomb and St. Clair Counties, Michigan
and
Assistant Professor of Pathology
Wayne State University School of Medicine
Detroit, Michigan

Jennifer Pierce-Weeks, RN, SANE-A, SANE-P
Forensic Nurse Examiner Program
Memorial Health System
Colorado Springs, Colorado

Kim Wieczorek, MSN, RN, SANE-A, SANE-P
Forensic Nurse Examiner
Forensic Nursing Program
St. Mary's Hospital
Richmond, Virginia

PHOTO CONTRIBUTORS*

Kathy Bell, MS, RN, SANE-A, SANE-P
Forensic Nursing Administrator
Tulsa Police Department
Tulsa, Oklahoma

Susan Chasson, MSN, JD, SANE-A
Family Nurse Practitioner
Merrill Gappmayer Family Medicine Center
and
Lecturer
College of Nursing
Brigham Young University
Provo, Utah

Renae Diegel, RN, BBL, CEN, CFN, CMI-III, D-ABMDI, SANE-A, CFC, DABFN, DABFE
Medical Examiner Investigator
Macomb County Medical Examiner's Office
Mt. Clemens, Michigan
and
Forensic Nurse Examiner/Educator
Turning Points Forensic Nurse Examiner Program
Clinton Township, Michigan

David Effron, MD, FACEP
Attending Physician
Department of Emergency Medicine
MetroHealth Medical Center
Cleveland, Ohio
and
Assistant Professor
Case Western Unversity
Cleveland, Ohio

Angie Ellis, BSN, RN, SANE-A, SANE-P, CEN
RN Manager-Forensic Nursing Services
Fairbanks Memorial Hospital
Fairbanks, Alaska

Tara Henry, MSN, FNP-C, SANE-A, SANE-P
Forensic Nurse Services
Anchorage, Alaska

Jennifer M. Meyer, RN, BSN, SANE-A, SANE-P
Clinical Nurse Manager
Forensic Nursing Services of Providence
Anchorage, Alaska

Valorie Prulhiere, BSN, RN, SANE-A
Coordinator of Victim Services
The DOVE Program
Summa Health System
Akron, Ohio

Linda Rossman, RN, MSN, WHNP-BC, PNP-BC, SANE-A, SANE-P
Manager: Nurse Examiner Program
YWCA West Central Michigan
Grand Rapids, Michigan

*The authors would also like to acknowledge the Department of Dermatology at Metrohealth Medical Center in Cleveland for granting permission for the use of some of their material.

REVIEWERS

Eileen M. Allen, MSN, RN, FN-CSA, SANE-A, SANE-P
SANE/SART Program Coordinator
Monmouth County Prosecutor's Office
Freehold, New Jersey
and
Adjunct Faculty
Monmouth University
West Long Branch, New Jersey

Connie Brogan, RN, CEN, SANE-A
Saint Luke's Health System
System Clinical Director Forensic Care Program
Kansas City, Missouri

Cathy Carter-Snell, RN, PhD, ENC-C, SANE-A
Associate Professor, Coordinator
Forensic Studies Program & Forensic Research
Network
Mount Royal University
Calgary, Alberta, Canada

Cari Caruso, RN, SANE-A
CEO Forensic Nurse Professionals, Consultant,
Educator
Forensic Nurse Professionals
Simi Valley, California

Denise S. Covington, MSN, RN, CEN, SANE-A
SAFE Program Coordinator
Office of Victim Services, Judicial Branch
Wethersfield, Connecticut

Sheila D. Early, RN, BScN, SANE-A
Coordinator, Forensic Health Sciences Option
Forensic Science and Technology
British Columbia Institute of Technology
Burnaby, British Columbia, Canada

Stephanie Eklund, MD, FACOG
Medical Director
Forensic Nursing Services of Providence
and
OB/Gyn department, Southcentral Foundation
Alaska Native Medical Center
Anchorage, Alaska

Christine (Cris) K. Finn, PhD, RN, FNP, FNE, MS, CEN, CFN, CPHQ
Assistant Professor
Regis University
Denver, Colorado

Carrie E. Huntsman-Jones, RN, MSN, CPN
Salt Lake SANE
Salt Lake City, Utah

Kathleen Sanders Jordan, RN, MS, FNB-BC, SANE-P
Nurse Practitioner at MidAtlantic Emergency
Medicine Associates
and
Lecturer at The University of North Carolina at
Charlotte
Mid-Atlantic Emergency Medicine Associates
Charlotte, North Carolina

Jennifer M. Meyer, RN, BSN, SANE-A, SANE-P
Clinical Nurse Manager
Forensic Nursing Services of Providence
Anchorage, Alaska

Christine Marie Michel, PhD, BSc, RN, DABFN
SANE Coordinator
Yukon-Kuskokwim Health Corporation
Bethel, Alaska

Stacey A. Mitchell, DNP, RN, SANE-A, SANE-P, D-ABMDI
Director, Forensic Nursing Services
Harris County Hospital District
Houston, Texas

Georgia A. Pasqualone, MSFS, MSFN, RN, CFN, CEN, FABFN
Adjunct Faculty
Boston College
Chestnut Hill, Massachusetts

Diana Schunn, RN, BSN, SANE-A, SANE-P
Executive Director
Child Advocacy Center of Sedgwick County
and
SANE/SART Specialist at Via Christi Health
Wichita, Kansas

Lynda M. Tiefel, BSN, RN, CEN, SANE-A
Forensic Nurse Examiner
Tiefel Legal Consulting
and
Refuge House Rape Crisis Program
Tallahassee, Florida

Elise J. Turner, MSN, CNM, SANE-A
Instructor
Hinds Community College
Raymond, Mississippi

The International Association of Forensic Nurses (IAFN) is an international membership organization composed of forensic nurses and other professionals who support and complement the work of forensic nursing. The mission of the IAFN is to provide leadership in forensic nursing practice by developing, promoting, and disseminating information internationally about forensic nursing science. IAFN recognized the need for an atlas with current evidence-based scientific information on adolescent and adult sexual assault that is a comprehensive, yet compact reference. With that in mind, IAFN created the *Atlas of Sexual Violence* to provide an illustrative overview of critical content associated with providing healthcare to patients affected by sexual violence. It is meant to be used as a tool for forensic clinicians who provide healthcare to adolescent and adult sexual assault patients. This book can also be invaluable to nurses and physicians from a variety of specialties, nursing and medical students, and other healthcare providers who utilize clinical photographs for learning, teaching, and practicing healthcare. Law enforcement, attorneys, criminalists, and other forensic professionals can benefit from this book by using it to enhance their knowledge and understanding of medical-forensic patient care and the role of forensic clinicians in the healthcare response to sexual violence.

More than 200 outstanding photographs are included in this book. Clinicians from forensic nurse examiner programs, emergency departments, and dermatology departments provided the collection of photographs. These clinical images are supported by evidence-based information that will assist the forensic clinician to diagnose, treat, and make referrals for injuries and dermatologic conditions identified during a sexual assault medical-forensic examination.

Chapter 1 discusses current practice standards for the healthcare response to sexual violence. Topics include the role of healthcare providers in sexual assault evaluations, physical and psychological assessment of the sexual assault patient, medical-forensic examination equipment and tools, forensic sample collection and preservation, and collaboration with multidisciplinary community partners.

Chapter 2 provides an overview of mechanisms of injury and injury terminology used in medical-forensic healthcare. Topics include blunt and sharp force injuries, patterned injuries, and defensive injuries. Narrative, diagrammatic, and photographic documentation are also discussed.

Chapter 3 reviews the anatomy and physiology of the body orifices penetrated in a sexual assault. Topics include male and female genitalia, anus, rectum, and oral cavity. Changes associated with puberty are also discussed.

Chapter 4 addresses common anogenital dermatological findings that may be seen during a sexual assault examination. Topics include skin anatomy, terminology of skin lesions, normal dermatologic variances, and a variety of infections. Practice implications for forensic clinicians are also reviewed.

Chapter 5 discusses current scientific evidence related to the presence and absence of injury from consensual intercourse. Topics include a literature review and clinical application for forensic clinicians.

Chapter 6 provides an overview of anogenital injury that may be seen during a sexual assault examination. Topics include injury prevalence, colposcope examination, toluidine blue dye, Foley catheter technique, digital and foreign body penetration, and oral penetration. Injuries in the adolescent and postmenopausal patient are also discussed.

Chapter 7 provides an overview of postmortem sexual assault examinations. To our knowledge, this is the first chapter ever produced with a comprehensive collection of colposcopic anogenital images from sex-related homicides. Topics include an overview of sex-related homicide, postmortem forensic sample collection, anogenital examination, postmortem changes, and anogenital injury.

Thank you to Elsevier for believing in this project. This book could not have been completed without the talented authors, photograph contributors, and reviewers. We thank you for the many hours of time and work you contributed to the creation of this *Atlas*.

Most of all, we thank the patients who gave their permission for their photographs to be taken and used for education purposes.

To the many forensic nurses, physicians, and other healthcare providers providing the healthcare response to sexual assault: Care deeply about your patients affected by sexual violence. It is an honor to be a forensic clinician helping those in need.

Tara Henry, MSN, FNP-C, SANE-A, SANE-P
Volume Editor

Carey Goryl, MSW, CAE
Chief Executive Officer
International Association of Forensic Nurses

TABLE OF CONTENTS

CHAPTER 1

CARE OF THE SEXUALLY ASSAULTED PATIENT

Susan Chasson and Kim Day

OVERVIEW OF SEXUAL ASSAULT AS A HEALTHCARE ISSUE

Sexual assault is a healthcare problem, requiring a healthcare response. According to the National Center for Victims of Crime, "sexual assault takes many forms, including attacks such as rape or attempted rape, as well as any unwanted sexual contact or threats." To formulate a response, it is important to understand the incidence and prevalence of sexual assault and the physical and psychological effects sexual violence has on victims. **Incidence** is the number of cases that occur in a period of time, while **prevalence** is the percentage of a population that has experienced an event at least once during a period of time (Kilpatrick, McCauley, 2009). Studies on sexual assault use many different approaches to look at incidence and prevalence, as well as multiple definitions for sexual assault, making it difficult to measure the extent of the problem (Kilpatrick, Ruggiero, 2004). Many victims never report their assault, so numbers generated by criminal justice programs are significantly lower than numbers reported by other types of surveys. Lifetime prevalence and annual incidence help in the understanding of the impact sexual assault has on victims as well as the overall healthcare system, and allows for a more accurate comparison to other healthcare issues.

In 2000, a national violence against women study approximated lifetime prevalence of sexual assault in the United States as 1 in 6 for women and 1 in 33 for men. Data from the study, in which 8000 women and 8005 men were interviewed, estimated that 302,091 women and 92,748 men were forcibly sexually assaulted in the United States in the year prior to the study (Tjaden, Thoennes, 2000). In some communities the rate is even higher, with American Indian/ Alaska Native women experiencing sexual assault at a rate greater than 1 in 3 (Amnesty International, 2007). These figures suggest that many, if not most, Americans have been impacted by sexual assault either personally, or by the effects of the assault on someone they know.

> The impact of sexual assault on a person's health is both immediate and long term.

In addition to any physical injury that a patient may have sustained at the time of the assault, the immediate impact can include unwanted pregnancies and sexually transmitted infections (STI). It is estimated that 5% of sexual assaults will result in an unwanted **pregnancy** (Holmes, Resnick, Kilpatrick, Best, 1996). Individuals who experience sexual assault can have short-term health problems such as sleep disturbances, change in appetite, and nightmares. Some of the long-term health consequences include drug and alcohol abuse, eating disorders, headaches, pelvic pain, abdominal pain, and fibromyalgia. Depression, anxiety and an increased risk for **suicide** can also result from sexual assault (Luce, 2010).

> Studies indicate that the impact of sexual assault and abuse can last a lifetime and reduces both the quality of life and life expectancy due to an increased risk of adverse health behaviors and outcomes that include drug and alcohol abuse, smoking, and obesity (Anda, Felitti, Bremmer, et al., 2006).

OVERVIEW OF SANE AND SART

Sexual Assault Nurse Examiners (SANE) as part of a **Sexual Assault Response Team** (SART) is a model of care developed about 30 years ago. Sexual assault is rather unique in terms of crimes in that the body of the living individual is considered one of the scenes of the crime. That victim's body must be investigated; much as any other crime scene would, requiring identification, documentation and collection of evidence. Types of evidence to obtain include documentation of injury, collection of secretions, hair or other types of debris, and trace evidence from the body.

> The intimate nature of the detailed medical-forensic evaluation, and the approach required to prevent re-traumatizing these patients, requires the skills of a specially trained healthcare provider.

Irrespective of their decisions to report sexual assault to legal authorities, victims of sexual assault often will seek medical care (World Health Organization

[WHO], 2003) further emphasizing the importance of healthcare in the response to sexual violence.

> The World Health Organization's position on the medical care of the sexual assault patient includes the following warning: "Performing a forensic examination without addressing the primary healthcare needs of the patient is negligent" (WHO, 2003, p 17).

Prior to the development of SANE practices, multiple studies documented the impact on victims who perceived their interactions with emergency department staff as upsetting and distressing and contributing to a feeling of being "re-raped" (Campbell, Sefl, Barnes, et al., 1999; Campbell, Wasco, Ahrens, et al., 2001; Ullman, 1996). The stark reality of this treatment for sexual assault patients in emergency departments prompted "pioneer" nurses in the 1970s to respond to this crisis by training registered nurses to provide comprehensive care to sexual assault patients (Lang, 1999; Ledray, 1999). These individuals were able to slowly impact their local systems and began a national movement toward using specially trained nurses to provide more patient-centered, compassionate care. It is a testament to these individuals' efforts that studies done in the decades following their work indicate that SANE programs have impacted the quality of patient care (Littel, 2001; Campbell, Patterson, Adams, et al., 2008; Plichta, Clements, Houseman, 2007; Fehler-Cabral, Campbell, Patterson, 2011) as well as criminal justice outcomes (WHO, 2002; Lenehan, 1991; Littel, 2001; Campbell, Bybee, Ford, Patterson, 2008).

Some of the acronyms that may be used to indicate healthcare professionals who have received specialized training to care for sexual assault patients include:

SANE: sexual assault nurse examiner

SAFE: sexual assault forensic examiner (may be a nurse, physician, or physician's assistant)

SAE: sexual assault examiner (may be a physician or physician's assistant)

FNE: forensic nurse examiner (a nurse who may see all types of forensic patients)

The positive impact of SANE programs is multi-faceted as gauged by numerous studies examining the effectiveness of SANEs.

> Patients treated by SANE programs describe experiences that demonstrate improved **psychological** well-being.

These experiences include feeling listened to, feeling safer, being given control, and being informed throughout the examination process, which results in reduced anxiety (Erikson, Dudley, McIntosh, et al., 2002; Campbell, Patterson, Lichty, 2005).

> The patients also experience improved healthcare outcomes with increased access to sexually transmitted infection (STI) prevention and treatment, emergency contraception, and physical assessments.

In addition to improved healthcare, studies indicate SANEs have fewer errors in evidence collection, more thorough sexual assault evidence kit collection, and improved documentation (Seivers, Murphy, Miller, 2003; Campbell, Patterson, Bybee, Dworkin, 2009). Realizing the positive impact of SANE programs, nurses and communities have embraced this model. As of April 2010, the **International Association of Forensic Nurses (IAFN)** *Clinical Program Registry* includes 553 clinical programs in the United States and 36 international programs. Although this represents a huge increase in programs, there are still regions of North America and many countries internationally that need inroads made in sexual assault medical-forensic examination program development.

When a person is a victim of sexual assault or abuse they may initially reach out to any number of community systems or agencies for a first response. Each one of these community agencies must be prepared to provide assurance to the victim that they are safe from further harm, and provide access to the resources they need to prevent or diminish the physical, psychological, and psychosocial consequences from the sexual assault. The *National Protocol for Sexual Assault Medical Forensic Examinations* notes that some form of a sexual assault response team is useful to coordinate immediate interventions and services (U.S. Department of Justice Office on Violence Against Women, 2004). These services may include: victim support, medical care, evidence collection and documentation, and the initial criminal investigation.

It is this emphasis on relationships with multiple agencies working together toward the common goal of assisting the sexual assault victim that has led to the formation of SART in the United States. These teams may also be referred to as Coordinated Community Response Teams (CCRT), Sexual Assault Resource and Response Teams (SARRT), or Multidisciplinary Teams. The general goal of the team is to assure a co-ordinated, victim-centered response to sexual assault at the local community level.

SARTs are composed of individuals who work with sexual assault victims at many levels in the community. They may include first responders such as Emergency Medical Systems (EMS), law enforcement, or rape crisis hotline team representatives. Community advocacy agencies who offer services for acute and long-term crisis intervention, medical accompaniment, and counseling services are often facilitators of the coordinated response and vital team members. SANE program staff, prosecutor's office representatives, and systems-based advocates are also included on most SARTs. Some teams also include forensic laboratory staff. Just as communities vary in location and diversity, it is important that SARTs reflect the unique characteristics of that community.

THE ROLE OF MEDICAL PROVIDERS IN SEXUAL ASSAULT EVALUATIONS

Sexual violence impacts the health and well-being of patients, families, and communities.

> It is essential that the medical care and treatment of patients provided in a compassionate, holistic manner is the underlying capstone of the medical-forensic examination, and consequently the primary role of the medical provider.

The *National Protocol for Sexual Assault Medical Forensic Examinations* defines the healthcare provider role in the care of the sexual assault patient as "providing compassionate and quality healthcare, collecting evidence in a thorough and appropriate manner, and testifying in court if needed" (U.S. Department of Justice Office on Violence Against Women, 2004). The examiner is a specially trained healthcare provider who can conduct the medical-forensic examination,

which includes: obtaining the medical and forensic history, performing a detailed physical assessment, collecting and preserving forensic evidence, providing treatment for injuries, prevention of sexually transmitted infections, and pregnancy risk evaluation and prevention.

The nursing care of the patient with the chief complaint of sexual assault or abuse begins with assessment, diagnosis, planning, intervention, and evaluation.

> The care of acute medical needs, and stabilization and treatment for life-threatening injuries, takes precedence over evidence collection.

The forensic consequences of any care provided should be considered and interventions documented by all healthcare providers who care for the patient prior to the medical-forensic examination.

Seeking informed consent from the patient for the medical-forensic evaluation is an integral component of the examination process. **Informed consent** is based on the concept that adults have the right to decide what happens to their bodies (Schloendorf vs. Society of New York Hospital, 1914).

> Informed consent should include verbal and written information about the examination, the risks, benefits, and alternatives to having a medical-forensic examination as well as possible consequences of not having an examination.

In the United States patients are assumed to give consent for the purposes of treatment in the case of life threatening emergencies. This is called **implied consent**. This is not the case for the medical-forensic examination, which is purely voluntary and not an emergency procedure. In addition to obtaining consent for the purpose of providing care, under federal privacy regulations created by the **Health Insurance Portability and Accountability Act (HIPAA)** patients are required to give written authorization for the purpose of releasing health information to someone who is not a healthcare provider such as law enforcement or a prosecutor (45 C.F.R. § 164.508). Sexual assault examiners should make sure their policies comply with both federal and state healthcare privacy laws. Policies should include procedures that address informed consent for patients who are adolescents, cognitively impaired, or unconscious (Pierce-Weeks, Campbell, 2008). It is important examiners recognize that during the sexual assault medical-forensic examination, consent is not a one-time event. Patients should be informed they may decline any portion of the medical-forensic examination and examiners should reassess consent throughout the examination process (U.S. Department of Justice Office on Violence Against Women, 2004). Criminal justice system participation and evidence collection is a voluntary process for the patient to choose or decline. The examiner should understand and be able to explain to the patient options for reporting the incident to criminal authorities. This includes explanation of any mandatory reporting laws.

Although providing healthcare is the primary role of the sexual assault examiner, throughout the examination process, the examiner is aware of the possibility that the case may be litigated in the criminal justice system. One of the advantages of SANE programs has been the willingness of examiners to testify in criminal and civil proceedings (Littel, 2001; Stone, Henson, Mclaren, 2006). SANE education includes emphasis on objective documentation of findings and understanding of courtroom procedures. This specialized training has increased the skills of nurses and the comfort level of the practitioner to testify to findings from the examination in the courtroom, and has demonstrated improved outcomes (Campbell, Patterson, Bybee, Dworkin, 2009).

One hallmark of the sexual assault examiner practice is interaction with the agencies that immediately respond to sexual assault. The primary collaboration at the time of the examination typically occurs between nurses, advocates, and law enforcement officers. Collaboration with victim advocates at the patient's bedside assures that the patient will have support through the examination and assistance with follow up to available community resources and criminal justice systems (if they have elected to report).

> Research has shown that when examiners work together with victim advocates, it enhances how victims perceive their overall care from both law enforcement and SANEs (Campbell, Patterson, Lichty, 2005).

The International Association of Forensic Nurses strongly supports collaboration between SANEs and advocates (International Association of Forensic Nurses, 2009). Collaboration with law enforcement for post-examination safety planning, release of the evidence, and discussing examination findings, enhances both patient care and criminal justice outcomes. Likewise, collaboration with other healthcare providers is another essential component of sexual assault care. Working with a program medical director to assure quality peer review, policy and protocol development, and facilitating healthcare provider follow-up in the community, will benefit patients (Ferrell, Awad, Markowitz, 2009).

ASSESSMENT OF THE SEXUAL ASSAULT PATIENT

It is important for the sexual assault patient to be evaluated in the same manner as any other patient. Assessment should involve both history taking and a physical assessment. Much as any patient encounter, the examination begins with the patient's chief complaint. This may vary from the patient reporting they are a victim of sexual assault, to reporting because they are unsure what has happened.

The initial assessment begins with a medical history that includes the following: allergies, medications, chronic physical and mental health problems, and previous surgeries. Risk for self-harm should be assessed. These categories provide a basis for asking further health questions in order to provide safe care to the patient. A medication list gives the healthcare provider an indication of any chronic health problems that may impact the physical or mental health of the patient. Chronic health problems potentially impact the care required by a sexual assault patient. For example, a patient who takes aspirin might need additional assessment to determine if they are at risk for either excessive bleeding or a clot formation after an assault. Previous surgeries may necessitate adaptation of the examination due to physical limitations (e.g., a patient whose spine has been surgically fused or one whose cervix has been removed due to hysterectomy). The history should also include details of the assault, and use of weapons, restraints, and forms of physical force, if used (Cantu, Coppola, Lindner, 2003). All patients should be asked about strangulation, including if they experienced loss of consciousness or bowel or bladder incontinence. Patients reporting strangulation may need to receive further evaluation to assess the potential for airway obstruction, which might be indicated if strangulation is accompanied by shortness of breath, behavioral changes, difficulty speaking or swallowing, or visible neck lesions (McClane, Strack, Hawley, 2001). The patient should also be asked if the assault was photographed or videotaped. This may have immediate psychological implications for the patient if photographs are taken during the examination, as well as longer term implications if the images taken by the assailant are distributed publicly.

If a patient reports unexplained loss of consciousness or decreased awareness, the examiner should make further inquiries about use of drugs and alcohol prior to the assault. Loss of consciousness in the absence of strangulation or head trauma may be an indication of drug- or alcohol-facilitated sexual assault and appropriate urine and blood samples should be collected for analysis. Information about personal hygiene following the assault, such as bathing or tooth brushing, may provide explanations for the presence or absence of the assailant's DNA.

> Information about the identity of the assailant should be obtained. If the assailant is known to the victim, it is important to determine if there is a risk of threat or injury to the patient after discharge (Markowitz, Steer, Garland, 2005).

The sexual assault examination should always be deferred if the patient has injuries or health problems that require immediate medical attention. The physical examination should be performed with a systematic approach that allows the examiner to evaluate each part of the patient's body, yet maintains the privacy and modesty of the patient. It begins with a head to toe examination of all body surfaces to look for injury. Palpation of the scalp should be performed to identify areas of tenderness or swelling. The oral cavity should be examined with attention given to the soft palate in cases of reported oral assault. Any jewelry or piercings should be inspected to look for evidence of trauma. Careful attention should be given to inspecting the

sclera and conjunctiva of strangulation victims to look for petechiae or hemorrhage. The examiner should also look for the presence of self-inflicted injuries created by the victim's attempt to remove the assailant's hands or arms from their neck.

After examining the patient for **non-genital injury**, the examiner should begin the anogenital examination. The **anogenital** examination may include the use of magnification or toluidine blue dye to increase the likelihood of injury visualization. (The use of a colposcope, digital imaging, and other visualization tools will be discussed in detail later in this chapter.)

PSYCHOLOGICAL NEEDS DURING THE EXAMINATION

In addition to a physical assessment, the emotional and psychological state of the patient should be assessed. This assessment should include the immediate mental state of the patient. Is the patient able to consent and cooperate with an examination? Is the patient mentally or cognitively impaired to a degree that they are unable to consent for an examination? Once a determination has been made about the ability of the patient to consent and cooperate with an examination, the examiner should assess the patient for problems that may impact the patient during the examination process and after discharge. Does the patient have a history of underlying mental problems that put them at risk for self-harm?

The response of the SANE to the sexual assault patient should be based on an understanding of the short-term emotional needs of the victim and the long-term psychological effects of sexual assault. It is important to understand that the actions, attitude, and approach to the patient by the examiner may impact the patient's ability to make a healthy adaptation after the assault. In one study, Erickson and colleagues (2002) interviewed patients two months after the assault and the patients described the following nursing interventions as beneficial to their experience: being treated as a whole person, being given control over all aspects of the examination, and being given information about both the examination and the healthcare impacts of the assault. Healthcare providers need to take a holistic approach to the needs of the patient, including offering the patient the option of a support person during the examination (which may be the victim advocate) and taking the time to meet their immediate physical needs, such as offering food or drink. Allowing the patient to set the pace of the examination and giving them permission to take breaks as needed is also helpful.

Providing anticipatory guidance about some of the physical and emotional responses to sexual assault prepares the patient for dealing with the emotional responses that occur after an assault.

> The nurse should perform an initial assessment of suicide risk and access mental health services for more extensive crisis evaluation if the patient is at risk for self-harm.

EQUIPMENT AND TOOLS UTILIZED

The healthcare professional who is caring for the sexual assault patient may use examination adjuncts during the medical-forensic examination. These tools help to identify areas where possible forensic evidence is located or allow for better visualization of anatomy or injury. The **colposcope** is a tool that can be used to enhance visualization of the anogenital structures with magnification and a light source. Colposcopes are equipped with imaging capabilities (Figure 1-1) and can be used to document findings through photography. Many programs have chosen to use digital cameras alone instead of colposcopes for the purpose of anogenital photographic documentation.

Toluidine blue dye (Figure 1-2) is a nuclear stain used in gynecology for detecting neoplasms. The dye binds to exposed cell nuclei, and can enhance the appearance of disturbances of the skin surface of the vulva in sexual assault examinations (Lauber, Souma, 1982). Normal vulvar skin does not contain nuclei; therefore, it cannot bind with the dye. However, when disruptions in the skin layers are present, the dye binds to the nuclei of underlying tissue cells. The binding of the dye is called "uptake" and can allow the examiner to have better visualization of some findings. Any break in the skin surface, whether it is caused by a

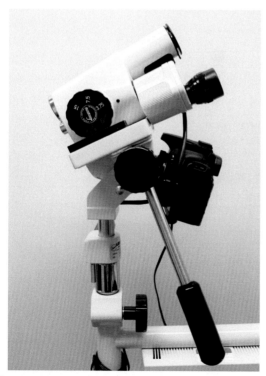

Figure 1-1
Colposcope with digital imaging capabilities.

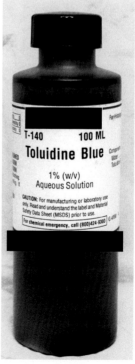

Figure 1-2
Toluidine blue dye 1% aqueous solution.

disease process or an injury, may "uptake" the dye if cell nuclei are exposed. Examiners should be trained in the application of toluidine blue dye and the interpretation of positive and negative "uptake" prior to its use.

The **sexual assault evidence collection kit** (also called a physical evidence recovery kit, evidence collection kit, forensic kit, or other local nomenclature) is another tool that is used during the medical-forensic examination (Figure 1-3). Although the contents of the evidence collection kit may vary by jurisdiction, in general the kit should contain an instruction sheet or checklist to guide the examiner through the collection procedure, and materials for collecting and preserving evidence (U.S. Department of Justice Office on Violence Against Women, 2004). Many standardized kits contain other supplies such as packaging materials and clothing bags, blood drawing supplies, blood stain card, paper drape, paper bindles, combs, swabs, and forms. The collection of evidence during the examination is guided by the scope of informed consent, the medical-forensic history, and local protocols.

A **speculum** is an instrument used to visualize the vagina and cervix. An **anoscope** is used to visualize the anal canal and rectum. These instruments may also facilitate the collection of evidence from these sites (Figure 1-4). In addition, the lower bill of the speculum may be used orally, in place of a tongue depressor, to observe for injury to the oral cavity. With this technique, the patient may be instructed to hold the speculum and apply downward pressure on their tongue. This allows the examiner to visualize the palate and posterior pharynx using light from the speculum (if equipped) or an external light source (Figures 1-5 and 1-6).

Digital cameras used during the examination vary by jurisdiction. In general, digital **photography** equipment has replaced the use of 35-mm and Polaroid photography equipment. Digital imaging is easy to use,

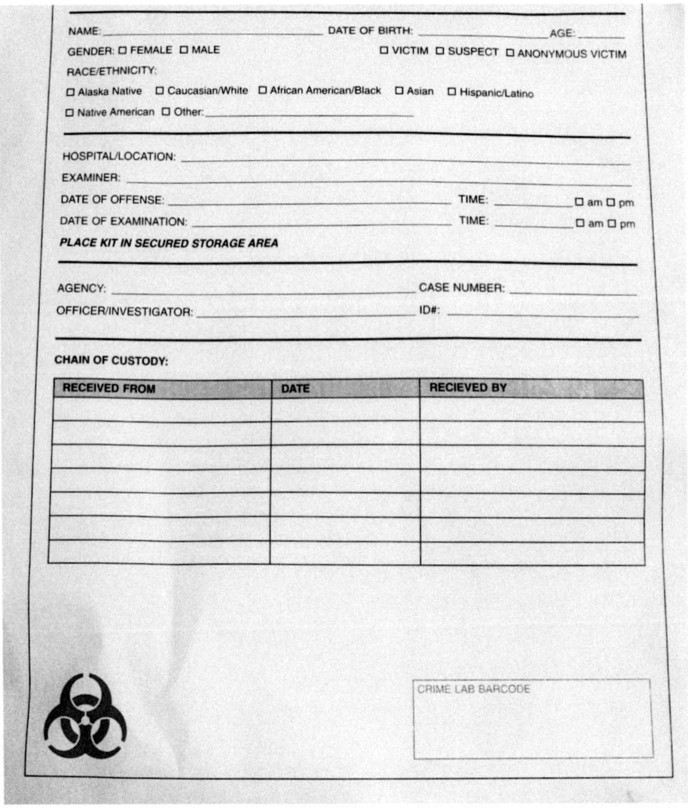

NAME: ____ DATE OF BIRTH: ____ AGE: ____

GENDER: ☐ FEMALE ☐ MALE ☐ VICTIM ☐ SUSPECT ☐ ANONYMOUS VICTIM

RACE/ETHNICITY:

☐ Alaska Native ☐ Caucasian/White ☐ African American/Black ☐ Asian ☐ Hispanic/Latino

☐ Native American ☐ Other: ____

HOSPITAL/LOCATION: ____

EXAMINER: ____

DATE OF OFFENSE: ____ TIME: ____ ☐ am ☐ pm

DATE OF EXAMINATION: ____ TIME: ____ ☐ am ☐ pm

PLACE KIT IN SECURED STORAGE AREA

AGENCY: ____ CASE NUMBER: ____

OFFICER/INVESTIGATOR: ____ ID#: ____

CHAIN OF CUSTODY:

RECEIVED FROM	DATE	RECIEVED BY

CRIME LAB BARCODE

Figure 1-3
Sexual assault evidence collection kit.

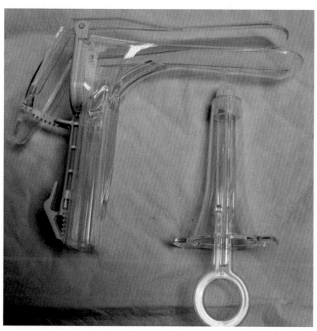

Figure 1-4
Plastic disposable speculum and anoscope.

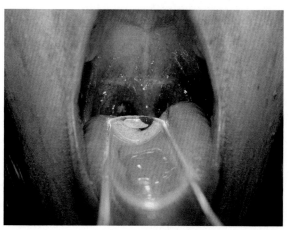

Figure 1-5
Visualization of the oral cavity using a speculum and light source.

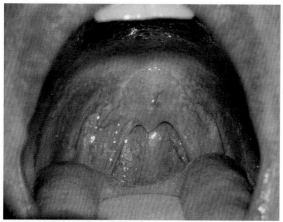

Figure 1-6
Visualization of the oral cavity using a tongue depressor and light source.

cost effective, and has eliminated the processing necessary with earlier photography methods. Digital cameras come with multiple features and accessories. Features to compare when purchasing a digital camera include: size of LCD screen (larger screen allows for better visualization during the examination), ability to use the camera with a power cord if the battery is drained, and the camera's time delay feature to facilitate taking images when both hands are needed during the examination. Many examiner programs have multiple users for the equipment, and should accommodate varying levels of expertise in photography.

Using appropriate lighting in the exam room is imperative to ensure the accurate capture of images. Having a quality macro lens allows for good close-up images of anatomical structures and the findings visualized by the nurse examiner. A tripod or monopod for camera stabilization and a remote control device to capture the photograph may also be helpful. The use of filters to highlight or enhance visualization of injury such as bruising or bite marks may also be helpful. The examiner must document the use of any filters used during the photography process.

Alternative Light Sources (ALS) with filter goggles may be used during the examination to identify possible sources of forensic evidence not apparent with direct visualization under standard examination room lighting. While the ALS can be used as a guide

to the location of possible substances on the skin (Figure 1-7), it cannot be used to positively identify semen (Carter-Snell, 2005). The ultraviolet light is indiscriminate and will fluoresce to many miscellaneous substances, and the nurse examiner must be aware of its limitations. The light source may not pick up significant substances and it may fluoresce insignificant substances.

FORENSIC SAMPLE COLLECTION AND PRESERVATION

Sources of potential forensic evidence are identified during the course of the medical-forensic examination.

> The history of the event will help guide the collection process and the use of a standardized sexual assault evidence collection kit will facilitate the preservation of forensic samples.

Timing considerations for evidence collection will vary by jurisdiction. Many jurisdictions collect forensic samples if the patient presents within three to five days of the reported assault. Those would be called "acute" exams. Examinations conducted beyond that period of time are called "non-acute" exams. Non-acute exams are beyond the window of opportunity to collect biological samples, but may be useful for evaluation of

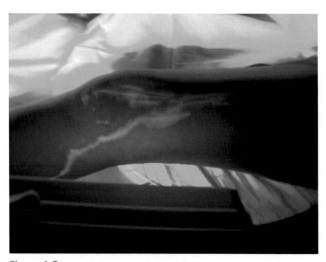

Figure 1-7
Fluorescence of dried fluid on leg seen using an alternative light source.

lingering injury. Environmental factors can affect the presence of evidence; therefore, examiners should take this into consideration when determining which forensic samples are to be collected. For example, if a patient has been immobilized or has been unable to bathe or perform hygiene activities, the time limitation for sample collection may be extended. Examiners should collaborate with forensic laboratory personnel who process sexual assault evidence kits, to ensure that techniques and collection methods are current with scientific research.

The types and location of evidence recovered can provide information about the nature of contact between individuals, as well as assist in the identification of the assailant. Specific techniques for evidence recovery may be used such as the double swab technique or wet-dry swabbing for the collection of bite mark samples. Currently, semen, blood, vaginal secretions, saliva, skin cells, and other biological materials can be processed and genetically identified by forensic laboratories. Although there are limitations on the ability to process certain sample types, advances in forensic science have improved to the point of needing only a few cells to produce forensic results. Following the scientific principles of forensic sample collection and preservation is imperative to ensure the samples collected during the examination are free from contamination and able to be processed by the forensic laboratory.

Clothing frequently contains evidence. Clothing worn by the patient during or immediately after the sexual assault should be collected and individually packaged for forensic lab analysis. Potential areas of evidence (e.g., alternative light source **fluorescence**, patient-identified area of ejaculate) should be documented and identified for the forensic lab. Items such as sanitary pads or tampons also are potentially rich sources of forensic materials. Special care should be taken to adequately dry and properly package these items to prevent degradation of the forensic sample. Policies should be in place to guide the examiner in drying of biological materials and clothing evidence or packaging for more definitive drying techniques.

Collection of forensic samples from the vagina, cervix, or rectum should be obtained prior to samples collected for medical screening tests. For example, if

the examiner's program routinely performs **sexually transmitted infection** testing for the sexual assault patient, the forensic samples should be collected prior. Collection of the anogenital swabs will be guided by the history of the assault and local protocol.

Specimens for toxicology will require urine and/or blood collection. Alcohol swabs should not be used to clean the area of withdrawal in the case of gray top tube collection for blood alcohol content. In the case of suspected drug- or alcohol-facilitated sexual assault, there may be additional forensic samples required. The examiner should be aware of requirements for laboratory specimen collection including type of sample, time frame, packaging, and transport. Some forensic laboratories may not process these specialized specimens on site; therefore, collaboration with the forensic laboratory to establish a process to address analysis of these samples is an important consideration.

DOCUMENTATION

Sexual assault medical-forensic examinations are performed by healthcare professionals; therefore, documentation should be consistent with other types of medical record documentation. Documentation should be objective, accurate, and complete. For example, instead of documenting "patient was upset," describe the behavior that was observed by the examiner, such as, "The patient was tearful at times." Statements made by the patient should be placed in quotation marks to indicate direct quotes reported by the patient to the examiner.

Many sexual assault examiners use standardized forms for the documentation of the medical-forensic examination. In addition to the medical history, most forms include questions about the history of the assault, history of drug or alcohol use prior to the assault, hygiene after the assault, and specific questions about sexual acts that occurred during the assault. Standardized forms also contain a list of samples collected during the examination including trace evidence, swabs, clothing, blood, and urine. The forms should include body diagrams to assist with documenting the location of genital and non-genital findings. Medications, immunizations, treatments, crisis interventions, and discharge instructions given during or after the examination should be documented in the medical record.

USE OF PHOTOGRAPHY AND IMAGE STORAGE

Examiners use photography to document genital and non-genital injury. At this time there is little evidence-based research surrounding the use of photography and its impact on either patient care or criminal justice outcomes (Sicchia, 2007).

> Photographs serve multiple purposes when taken as part of the sexual assault examination. They document the presence or absence of injury, provide opportunities for peer review and consultation, and can be used for educating new providers (Creighton, Alderson, Brown, Minto, 2002; Ernst, Speck, Fitzpatrick, 2011).

Examiners who use photography must have a clear understanding of why they are taking images. Informed consent from the patient should cover all anticipated use of photographs. Since images are being taken as part of a medical examination, they are considered to be part of the medical record. Release of images should take place only with written authorization from the patient and in compliance with any federal and state privacy laws (45 C.F.R. § 164.508, 2010).

Examiners should have a policy that describes the proper procedure for taking, storing, and releasing images. With increased use of digital photography and camera memory cards that allow hundreds of photographs to be stored on a single device, it important that a procedure is established to make sure the images from a single patient can be properly identified. Some examiners photograph a label with information that identifies the patient, followed by a facial image of the patient. After the photographs have been taken, the examiner places another photograph of the label to clearly mark the end of the series. Other examiners have an identification number that is included as part of the image file along with the date. It is important for the examiner to be able to state they were present when an image was made, and that the image is an accurate representation, or not, of what the examiner observed at the time of the exam (Shaw, 2002). The examiner should be able to describe the procedure for making sure photographs are properly identified as belonging to the correct patient.

One set of images should be stored with the patient's medical record. Some facilities create a backup of the original photos to be kept in a separate location. It is important that backup copies are maintained in a fashion that permits accessibility to the images as technology changes. Another important security consideration is the preservation and accessibility of images if there is a disaster such as a flood or fire. As clinical sites begin to use electronic medical records for sexual assault records, limiting access of sexual assault medical records and images to members of the sexual assault medical team should be considered (Rothstein, 2010).

Photographs used to document injury on the body should include three images for each injury when possible. The first image should be taken at a distance sufficient to indicate location on the body (Figure 1-8A). The second image should be a medium range of the actual injury (Figure 1-8B) and a third image should be a close-up that includes a measuring device to provide scale (Figure 1-8C). A photograph log can be created at the time of the exam to describe the location of the injury documented in each image.

Some jurisdictions may use the photographs from a sexual assault examination in the courtroom. The sensitive nature of the photographs, especially the anogenital photographs, makes any kind of disclosure a potential concern for the patient and the examiner. Examiners and their medical facility should establish protocols with law enforcement, prosecution, and defense attorneys to limit access to, and protect the images from, unauthorized distribution.

SEXUALLY TRANSMITTED INFECTIONS

It is difficult to accurately estimate the risk of exposure to a sexually transmitted infection (STI) after sexual assault (Reynolds, Peipert, Collins, 2000). While some STIs are preventable or treatable with medications or immunization, the herpes simplex viruses, hepatitis C virus, and the Human papillomavirus do not have effective methods of prophylaxis. Most sexual assault programs offer antibiotic prophylaxis to patients for the prevention of gonorrhea and chlamydia.

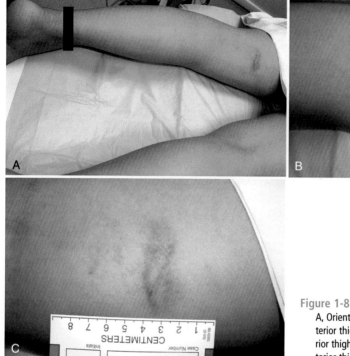
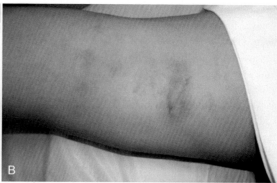

Figure 1-8
A, Orientation photograph showing location of bruising on left posterior thigh. B, Medium range photograph of bruising on left posterior thigh. C, Photograph with scale measuring bruising on left posterior thigh.

The Centers for Disease Control and Prevention (2010), provides a recommended protocol for STI prophylaxis after sexual assault.

This protocol may be altered by different programs depending on prevalence of certain infections. For example, if there is a low rate of trichomoniasis infection in the community, the risk of adverse affects when using Metronidazole, may be outweighed by the benefits of providing prophylactic treatment. Some programs may also find it difficult to provide hepatitis B immunization if they are not located in a facility that has the ability to store the hepatitis B immunization, and will refer their patients to local health departments or primary care providers for hepatitis B immunization.

The decision to perform STI testing at the time of the medical-forensic examination should be made based on the healthcare needs of the patient and the public health needs of the community. In communities where there is a high prevalence (Forhan, Gottlieb,

Sternberg, et al., 2009), testing may provide an opportunity to prevent the spread of sexually transmitted infections within the community. Testing considerations should include ability to follow up with the patient to provide test results and initiate partner treatment and the availability and cost of testing. A positive result at the time of the exam must be properly interpreted by the examiner since DNA-based testing for STIs may test positive in the presence of infected semen in a female patient (Holmes, 1999). It is important that STI medications be provided to patients at the time of the examination to increase rates of compliance after assault.

HUMAN IMMUNODEFICIENCY VIRUS (HIV) PROPHYLAXIS AFTER SEXUAL ASSAULT

In 2005, the Centers for Disease Control published recommendations for Non-occupational Post-exposure Prophylaxis for **human immunodeficiency virus** (HIV). The guidelines are clear that prophylaxis is indicated when there is a high risk exposure from a known HIV positive source. Unfortunately, most victims of sexual assault do not know if their assailant is positive for HIV. It is essential for all providers who care for sexual assault patients to have screening and treatment protocols in place for patients who are at risk for HIV. In addition to protocols, appropriate access to medications should be readily available to offer patients who need to start HIV prophylaxis. HIV prophylaxis should be started no later than 72 hours after possible exposure.

Informed consent should include information about the risk of obtaining an HIV infection related to the type of sexual contact, the risks related to known history of the assailant, and the risks associated with taking the medication for one month. The types of contact that demonstrate the highest risk for HIV transmission include sharing of needles, receptive anal intercourse, and receptive vaginal intercourse from a known HIV positive source. Individuals who are at increased risk for HIV infection include men who have sex with men, intravenous drug users, and assailants with a history of incarceration or with known hepatitis C infections (Wieczorek, 2010).

Protocols for HIV prophylaxis should incorporate procedures for informed consent, requirements for baseline lab testing, establishment of a medication regime, and should incorporate a program to provide patient follow-up. Baseline lab testing should include a pregnancy test (female victims of reproductive age), baseline tests for the HIV serology, liver function tests, and a complete blood count (CBC). Selection of a medication regime should occur in collaboration with HIV healthcare providers and the local health department. Medication for nausea should be included with HIV prophylaxis. Due to the limited availability of some anti-retroviral medications in small communities, a three- to five-day starter pack of medications should be provided to patients when prophylaxis is indicated. Patients should be given clear instructions for follow-up that include potential adverse reactions, contact information for the follow-up provider and an appointment for care (Wieczorek, 2010).

REPRODUCTIVE HEALTHCARE ISSUES PREGNANCY PREVENTION

Emergency contraception is the provision of contraceptive methods in the first few days after unprotected intercourse. Although methods for emergency contraception may vary, the most common and safest form of emergency contraception in use is levonorgestrel, a progestin hormone. It is sold in the United States under the brand name of **Plan B**. Many professional organizations have taken positions on the provision of emergency contraception in sexual assault (World Health Organization, 2003; American College of Obstetricians and Gynecologists, 2010; International Association of Forensic Nurses, 2009; American College of Emergency Physicians, 2008; U.S. Conference of Catholic Bishops, 2001). These position statements support immediate access to emergency contraception for all victims of sexual violence who choose to use it. Many states in the United States have enacted laws that require emergency facilities to offer emergency contraception to victims of sexual assault, yet there continues to be a lack of understanding about the mechanisms of action for emergency contraception among some healthcare providers.

> All medical facilities that treat patients who have been victims of sexual assault must have policies in place to address pregnancy risk evaluation and prevention.

Becoming pregnant as a result of sexual assault is a significant concern for patients. The risk of pregnancy from sexual assault is estimated to be between 2% and 5%, similar to that of a single act of unprotected intercourse. It is important to understand that the patient may have beliefs regarding acceptable treatment options for pregnancy prevention, and the examiner must be sensitive to those beliefs. Most programs offer pregnancy prevention methods for patients when they are seen within 120 hours of the assault. The examiner should be knowledgeable about the mechanisms of action of emergency contraception and be able to share that knowledge in a manner that is understandable to the patient. All emergency contraception options available should be objectively explained, without placing pressure on the patient.

FOLLOW-UP EXAMINATIONS

Follow-up visits help to facilitate the medical care and treatment of the patient beyond just the initial examination.

A follow-up examination provides an opportunity for the examiner to follow injury progression (Figure 1-9), assess resolution of injury (Figure 1-10), assist in identifying normal variances of initial findings (Figure 1-11), and allows for identification of additional physical manifestations related to the sexual assault that require referrals to a primary care provider for management.

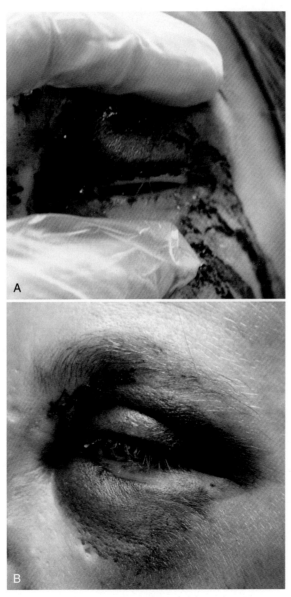

Figure 1-9
  A, Bruising and swelling left eye 3 hours after assault. B, Bruising and swelling left eye 36 hours after assault.

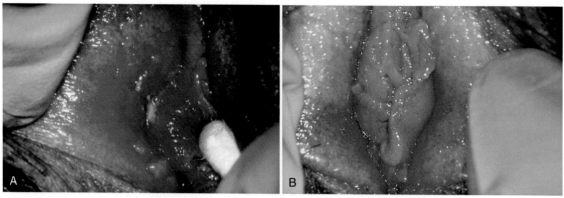

Figure 1-10

A, Bruising and swelling of hymen at initial examination 8 hours after assault. Redness on the labia minor is also visible. B, Resolution of bruising and swelling of hymen at follow-up examination 2 weeks after assault.

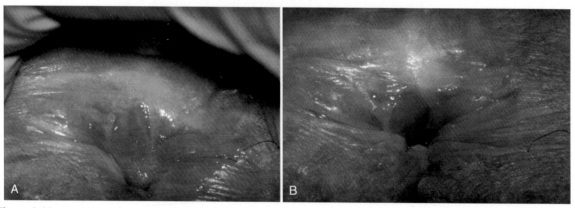

Figure 1-11

A, Chronic fissure at the 12 o'clock position on anus at initial examination 7 hours after assault. B, Chronic fissure at the 12 o'clock position on anus still present at follow-up examination one month after assault. This finding should not be confused with an acute laceration.

> A follow-up visit a few weeks after the initial examination provides an opportunity to reassess the short-term psychological and social sequelae of the sexual assault and provide intervention or referrals for the patient's identified needs.

Anticipatory guidance on possible physical and psychological signs and symptoms related to the sexual assault and a list of referral options for healthcare providers the patient can follow up with, if needed, should be provided at the initial examination.

The patient should be referred to primary healthcare providers to provide longer term care for follow-up STI testing, medication management in the case of HIV prophylaxis and monitoring for pregnancy if the patient declines pregnancy prophylaxis. Referral to mental health providers, rape crisis, and community based advocacy services for counseling and assistance should also be part of the plan of care for patients.

Key Terms

Alternative light source
Anogenital
Anoscope
Colposcope
Digital camera
Emergency contraception
Fluorescence
Health Insurance Portability and Accountability Act (HIPAA)
Human immunodeficiency virus (HIV)

Implied consent
Incidence
Informed consent
International Association of Forensic Nurses (IAFN)
Non-genital injury
Photography
Plan B
Prevalence
Psychological
Sexual assault evidence collection kit
Sexual assault nurse examiner (SANE)
Sexual assault response team (SART)
Sexually transmitted infection
Speculum
Suicide
Toluidine blue dye

References

American College of Emergency Physicians. (2008, October). *Management of the patient with the complaint of sexual assault.* Retrieved January 10, 2010, from http://www.acep.org/Content.aspx?id=29562&terms=sexual%20assault

American College of Obstetricians and Gynecologists. (May 2010). ACOG practice bulletin no. 112: Emergency contraception. *Obstetrics and Gynecology, 115,* 1100–1109.

Amnesty International. (2007). *Maze of injustice: The failure to protect indigenous women from sexual violence in the USA.* New York: Amnesty International.

Anda, R., Felitti, V., Bremmer, et al. (2006). The enduring effects of abuse and related adverse experiences in childhood: A convergence of evidence from neurobiology and epidemiology. *European Archives Psychiatry and Neuroscience 256*(3), 174–186.

Campbell, R., Bybee, D., Ford, J., & Patterson, D. (2008). *Systems change analysis of SANE programs: Identifying the mediating mechanisms of criminal justice system impact.* Retrieved January 10, 2010, from http://www.ncjrs.gov/pdffiles1/nij/grants/226497.pdf

Campbell, R., Patterson, D., Adams, A. E., et al. (2008). A participatory evaluation project to measure SANE nursing practice and adult sexual assault patients' psychological well-being. *Journal of Forensic Nursing, 4*(1), 19–28.

Campbell, R., Patterson, D., Bybee, D., & Dworkin, E. (2009). Predicting sexual assault prosecution outcomes. *Criminal Justice and Behavior, 36*(7), 712–727.

Campbell, R., Patterson, D., & Lichty, L. (2005). The effectiveness of sexual assault nurse examiner (SANE) programs: A review of psychological, medical, legal and community outcomes. *Trauma, Violence & Abuse, 6*(4), 313–329.

Campbell, R., Sefl, T., Barnes, H.E., et al. (1999). Community services for rape survivors: Enhancing psychological

well-being or increasing trauma? *Journal of Consulting and Clinical Psychology, 67,* 847–858.

Campbell, R., Wasco, S., Ahrens, C., et al. (2001). Preventing the "second rape": Rape survivors' experiences with community service providers. *Journal of Interpersonal Violence, 16,* 1239–1259.

Cantu, M., Coppola, M., & Lindner, A. (2003). Evaluation and management of the sexually assaulted woman. *Emergency Medicine Clinics of North America, 21,* 737–750.

Carter-Snell, C. S. (2005). Forensic ultraviolet lights in clinical practice: Evidence for the evidence. *Canadian Journal of Police and Security Services, 3*(2), 79–85.

Centers for Disease Control. (2005). Antiretroviral postexposure prophylaxis after sexual, injection-drug use, or other nonoccupational exposure to HIV in the United States. *Morbidity and Mortality Weekly Report, 54.*

Centers for Disease Control and Prevention. (2010). Sexually transmitted disease treatment guidelines. Retrieved May 1, 2011, from http://www.cdc.gov/std/treatment/2010/toc.htm

Creighton, S., Alderson, J., Brown, S., & Minto, C. (2002). Medical photography ethics, consent and the intersex patient. *British Journal of Urology, 89*(1), 67–72.

Erikson, J., Dudley, C., McIntosh, G., et al. (2002). Client's experience with specialized sexual assault service. *Journal of Emergency Nursing, 28*(1), 86–90.

Ernst, E., Speck, P., & Fitzpatrick, J. (2011). Usefulness of forensic photography after sexual assault. *Advanced Emergency Nursing Journal, 33*(1) 29–38.

Fehler-Cabral, G., Campbell, R., & Patterson, D. (2011, May 20). Adult sexual assault survivors' experiences with sexual assault nurse examiners. *Journal of Interpersonal Violence.* Retrieved June 15, 2011, from http://jiv.sagepub.com/content/early/2011/05/10/0886260511403761

Ferrell, J., Awad, S., & Markowitz, J. (2009). *Fostering collaboration between SANE program coordinators and medical directors.* Retrieved 2011 from VAWnet website: http://www.vaw.umn.edu/documents/SANECollaboration/SANECollaboration.pdf

Forhan, S., Gottlieb, S., Sternberg, et al. (2009). Prevalence of sexually transmitted infections among female adolescents aged 14–19 in the United States. *Pediatrics, 124,* 1505–1512.

Holmes, M. (1999). Sexually transmitted infections in female rape victims. *AIDS Patient CARE and STDs, 13*(12), 703–708.

Holmes, M., Resnick, H., Kilpatrick, D., & Best. C. (1996). Rape-related pregnancy: Estimates and descriptive characteristics from a national sample of women. *American Journal of Obstetricians and Gynecology, 175*(2), 320–324.

International Association of Forensic Nurses. (November, 2008). Postion statement: Collaboration with victim advocates. Retrieved May 1, 2011, from http://www.iafn.org/associations/8556/files/IAFN%20Position%20Statement-Advocate%20Collaboration%20Approved.pdf

International Association of Forensic Nurses. (October, 2009). Position statement: Use of emergency contraception post sexual assault. Retrieved May 1, 2011, from http://www.iafn.org/associations/8556/files/IAFN%20 Position%20Statement-Emergency%20Contraception%20 Approved.pdf

Kilpatrick, D., & McCauley, J. (2009). Understanding national rape statistics. *National Online Resource Center on Violence Against Women.* Retrieved May 1, 2011, from VAWnet website: http://www.vawnet.org/Assoc_Files_ VAWnet/AR_RapeStatistics.pdf

Kilpatrick, D., & Ruggiero, K. (2004). *Making sense of rape in America: Where do the numbers come from and what do they mean.* Retrieved 2010, from VAWnet website: http://www. vawnet.org/Assoc_Files_VAWnet/MakingSenseofRape.pdf

Lang, K. (1999). *Sexual assault nurse examiner resource guide for Michigan communities.* Okemos, MI: Michigan Coalition against Domestic and Sexual Violence.

Lauber, A., & Souma, M. (1982). Use of toluidine blue for documentation of traumatic intercourse. *Obstetrics and Gynecology, 60*(5), 644–648.

Ledray, L. (1999). *Sexual assault nurse examiner (SANE) development and operations guide.* Washington, DC: U.S. Department of Justice Office of Justice Programs for Victims of Crime.

Lenehan, G. (1991). Commentary: Sexual assault nurse examiners: A SANE way to care for rape victims. *Journal of Emergency Nursing, 17*(4), 190.

Littel, K. (2001). Sexual assault nurse examiner (SANE) programs: Improving the community response to sexual assault victims. Washington, DC: U.S. Department of Justice Office of Justice Programs for Victims of Crime.

Luce, H. S. (2010). Sexual assault of women. *American Family Physician, 81*(4), 489–495.

Markowitz, J., Steer, S., & Garland, M. (2005). Hospital-based intervention for intimate partner violence victims: A forensic nursing model. *Journal of Emergency Nursing, 81*(4), 489–495.

McClane, G., Strack, G., & Hawley, D. (2001). A review of 300 attempted strangulation cases: Part II clinical evaluation of the surviving victim. *Journal of Emergency Medicine, 21*(3), 311–315.

Pierce-Weeks, J., & Campbell, P. (2008). The challenge forensic nurses face when their patient is comatose: Addressing the needs of our most vulnerable patient population. *Journal of Forensic Nursing, 4,* 104–110.

Plichta, S., Clements, P., & Houseman, C. (2007). Why SANEs matter: Models of care for sexual violence victims in the emergency department. *Journal of Forensic Nursing, 3*(1), 15–23.

Reynolds, M., Peipert, J., & Collins, B. (2000). Epidemiologic issues of sexually transmitted diseases in sexual assault victims. *Obstetric and Gynecologic Survey, Jan 55*(1), 51–57.

Rothstein, M. (2010). The Hippocratic bargain and health information technology. *Journal of Law Medicine and Ethics, 38,* 7.

Schloendorff v. Society of N. Y. Hospital, 105 N.E. 93 (N.Y. 1914).

Seivers, V., Murphy, S., & Miller, J. (2003). Sexual assault evidence collection more accurate when completed by sexual assault nurse examiners: Colorado's experience. *Journal of Emergency Nursing, 29,* 511–514.

Shaw, C. (2002). Admissibility of digital photographic evidence: Should it be any different than traditional photography? *Update.* Alexandria, VA: American Prosecutors Research Institute.

Sicchia, S. (2007). *Colposcopy and anogenital photography in adult survivors of sexual assault.* Ontario Network of Sexual Assault and Domestic Violence Treatment Centers.

Stone, W., Henson, V., & McLaren, J. (2006). Law enforcement perceptions of sexual assault nurses in Texas. *The Southwest Journal of Criminal Justice, 3*(2), 103–126.

Tjaden, P., & Thoennes, N. (2000). *Full report of the prevalence, incidence and consequences of violence against women.* Washington, DC: U.S. Department of Justice Office of Justice Programs.

Ullman, S. (1996). Do social reactions to sexual assault victims vary by support provider? *Violence and Victims, 11*(2), 142–156.

United States Code of Federal Regulations. 45 C.F.R. § 164.508 (2010). Retrieved June 11, 2011, from http:// frwebgate.access.gpo.gov/cgi-bin/get-cfr.cgi?TITLE=45 &PART=164&SECTION=508&TYPE=TEXT

U.S. Conference of Catholic Bishops. (2001). Ehical and religious directive for healthcare services (4th ed., no. 36). Retrieved May 1, 2001, from http://www.usccb.org/bishops/ directives.shtml

U.S. Department of Justice Office on Violence Against Women. (2004). *A national protocol for sexual assault medical forensic examinations adults/adolescents.* Washington, DC: U.S. Department of Justice Office on Violence Against Women.

Wieczorek, K. (2010). A forensic nursing protocol for initiating human immunodeficiency virus post-exposure prophylaxis following sexual assault. *Journal of Forensic Nursing, 6*(1), 29–39.

World Heath Organization. (2002). *World report on violence and health.* Geneva: World Heath Organization. Retrieved May 1, 2011, from http://www.who.int/violence_injury_ prevention/violence/world_report/en/

Word Health Organization. (2003). *Guidelines for medicolegal care for victims of sexual violence.* Geneva: World Health Organization. Retrieved May 1, 2011, from http:// whqlibdoc.who.int/publications/2004/924154628X.pdf

CHAPTER 2

WOUND IDENTIFICATION AND DOCUMENTATION

Renae Diegel, Tara Henry, and Daniel J. Spitz

Conducting a medical-forensic examination on a patient seen for sexual assault involves completing a detailed head-to-toe evaluation.

> Wound assessment is a critical component of the diagnosis and treatment of forensic patient care.

To accurately identify body surface injuries, a forensic examiner must have an extensive knowledge of wound definitions, wound characteristics, and mechanisms of injury. They must also have a comprehensive understanding of how location, medications, infection, diseases or health conditions, and the patient's ability to care for the wound affect the healing process.

Forensic examiners should not attempt to determine how many hours or days old a wound is. Forensic examiners should have an understanding of the pathophysiology of the normal wound healing process and factors that may complicate it. Therefore, when assessing a wound, the forensic examiner must determine the following: if the wound may require repair; if imaging should be performed; how the wound should be cleaned; what type of dressing is required, if any; if pain relief is required; whether the patient requires a tetanus immunization; if any antibiotics need to be administered; if there may be any disruptions to the healing status; if the patient has co-morbidities; if a referral for additional evaluation is needed; and what type of wound care instructions a patient may require upon discharge.

This chapter will focus on injury terminology, mechanisms of injury, and the type of documentation that should be used in the medical-forensic evaluation of patients reporting a sexual assault. Blunt and sharp force trauma, patterned injuries, and defensive injuries will be discussed, as well as narrative, diagrammatic, and photographic methods of documentation.

BLUNT FORCE TRAUMA

Blunt force trauma is caused by impact to the body and probably is the single most common cause of trauma (Spitz, 2006). Blunt force injuries fall into four categories, which include bruises (contusions), abrasions (scratches and scrapes), lacerations (tears of the skin) and skeletal fractures. The severity and appearance of blunt traumatic injuries depend on the amount of force used, the area of the body struck, the time over which the force is delivered, and the characteristics of the weapon (Di Maio, Di Maio, 2001).

> **Bruises (contusions)** occur when an impact causes blood vessels to rupture and blood seeps into the surrounding tissues. This usually occurs when the skin is crushed or overstretched causing tearing of blood vessels and an escape of red blood cells into the tissue.

Bruises go through several stages of healing, and during this process their color and size change. Recent or fresh bruises are usually red to blue to purple in color, have well-defined margins (Figures 2-1 to 2-5),

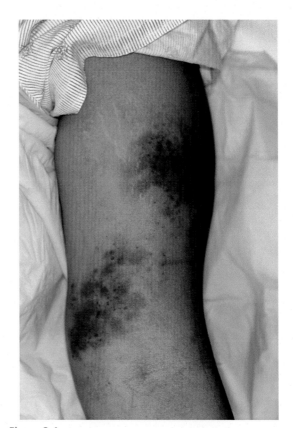

Figure 2-1
Red-purple bruising with well-defined margins on left upper arm.

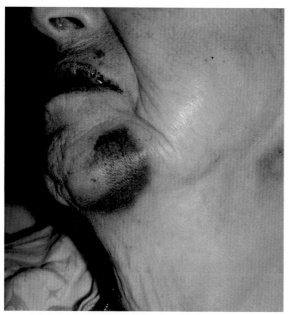

Figure 2-2
Blue-purple bruising with well-defined margins on chin.

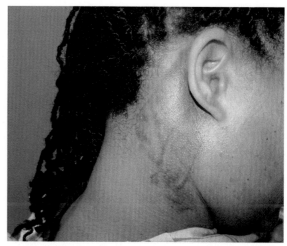

Figure 2-3
Red-purple bruising with well-defined margins over mastoid and right lateral neck.

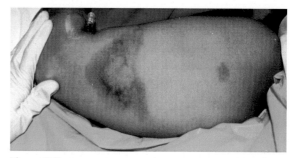

Figure 2-5
Red-blue-purple bruising with well-defined margins on left upper arm.

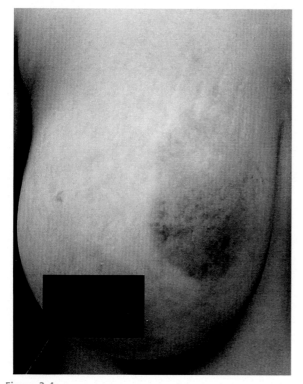

Figure 2-4
Red-purple bruising with well-defined margin on right breast.

and are often associated with pain and swelling. As bruises begin to heal, the color changes to green, yellow, and brown; margins fade; (Figures 2-6 to 2-10) and the pain and swelling resolve. Forensic examiners should have an understanding of the pathophysiology of bruise healing and color changes associated with each stage.

The color changes of a bruise are related to the inflammatory healing process. The release of red blood cells and **hemoglobin** into the tissue results in a reddish color, with blue to purple a result of further extravasation of venous blood into the tissue. During the inflammatory reaction, **macrophages** ingest the **erythrocytes** and hemoglobin metabolization begins. Hemoglobin is metabolized to biliverdin, which is responsible for the green color of a bruise. Yellowing of a bruise occurs when **biliverdin** converts to **bilirubin**. As iron degrades after its release from hemoglobin, the brown pigmentation of a bruise appears (Yajima, Funayama, 2006; Nash, Sheridan, 2009; Hughes, Ellis, Burt, Langlois, 2004; Langlois, 2007).

The color of a bruise and the rate at which it heals depends on many factors. Force of the impact, amount of blood released at the time of injury, location of bruise, thickness of skin, amount of subcutaneous tissue, patient's age, medications, and the overall health of the patient are several factors that influence bruising. Consensus has yet to be reached on the time frame between color changes of a bruise (Langlois,

2007). The perception of a bruise color can be affected by the skin tone of the person, the observer's ability to perceive color, lighting conditions used to view the bruise, and whether the bruise is viewed in person or by photograph (Nash, Sheridan, 2009; Langlois, 2007; Yajima, Funayama, 2006; Hughes, Ellis, Langlois, 2004). Opinions regarding the age of a bruise, stated in hours or days, should not be attempted by forensic examiners due to the numerous factors that affect the presence or absence of a bruise, healing stages, and visibility of color.

Opinions that are given related to bruising should rely on the patient's history, characteristics of the bruise, and a thorough understanding of the pathophysiology of bruising and current associated research.

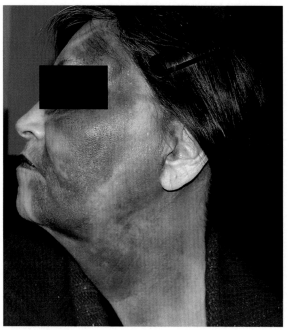

Figure 2-7
Purple-yellow-green bruising with faded margins on face and neck.

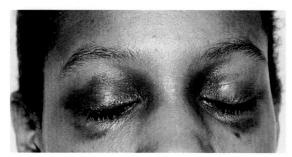

Figure 2-6
Red-yellow periorbital bruising with faded margins.

Bruises are not always visible immediately; however, they are oftentimes preceded by pain at the injured location. Therefore, body surfaces without visible injury must still be assessed for pain and palpated for tenderness or swelling. When indicated, a 24- to 48-hour follow-up examination should be arranged to assess for bruises that may have evolved.

Petechiae are a form of bruising that results from rupture of capillaries, the body's smallest blood vessels.

Rupture can occur from blunt impact or from an increase in internal capillary pressure. Ruptured capillaries from increased internal capillary pressure are

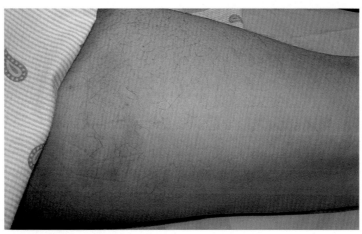

Figure 2-8
Red-yellow-brown bruising with faded margins on left thigh.

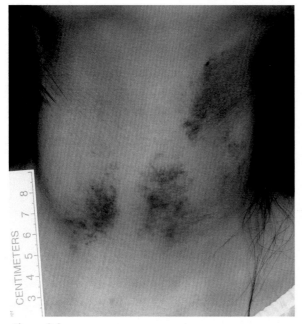

Figure 2-9
Purple-yellow bruising with fading margins on neck.

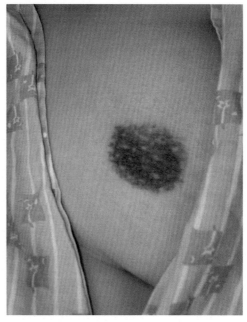

Figure 2-10
Red-yellow bruising with fading margins on left breast.

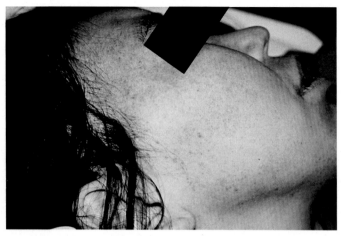

Figure 2-11
Confluent petechiae on face.

often seen on the face and conjunctiva from incidences such as strangulation, vomiting, severe coughing, or pushing during the second stage of labor. Petechiae are red, non-elevated, less than 3 mm in diameter, and can be a singular capillary rupture or multiple (Figure 2-11).

Ecchymosis is frequently misdiagnosed by clinicians. Clinicians have often used ecchymosis and bruise as interchangeable terms; however, there are differences that should be understood to ensure proper terminology is used.

Ecchymosis is often used to describe the blue-purple hemorrhagic areas that are common on the hands and forearms of the elderly (senile ecchymosis).

Ecchymosis is a non-elevated, painless, hemorrhagic spot, which typically appears as a non-patterned blue, black or purplish patch (Figure 2-12). It is induced by bleeding of a hematological nature and is not the result of trauma to the body (Besant-Matthews, 2011).

Care should be taken when describing such findings. Although these lesions may be the result of spontaneous bleeding secondary to an underlying hematological condition, often they are exacerbated by minor trauma in the elderly; therefore, the distinction between bruising and ecchymosis in this situation is not always clear.

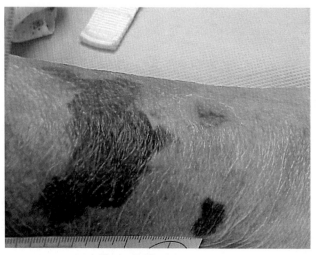

Figure 2-12
Ecchymosis on right arm.

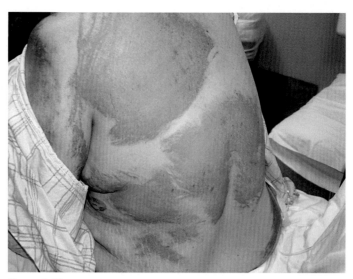

Figure 2-13
Abrasions on back.

An **abrasion** is caused by the rubbing or scraping away of the superficial layer of skin from a mechanical means such as blunt impact.

Abrasions are typically confined to the epidermal and dermal layers of skin and do not involve the deeper tissue (Figure 2-13). Abrasions caused by blunt impact may occur in conjunction with a contusion (Figures 2-14 and 2-15). Abrasions are of great importance because they reveal the exact point of contact between an object and the body. They often allow for the determination of the mechanism of injury as well as indicate the direction of the force. Recognizing a patterned abrasion can be helpful in the identification of the object used to create the injury.

Lacerations are caused by an impact that results in tearing, ripping, crushing, overstretching or shearing of soft tissue (Besant-Matthews, 2011).

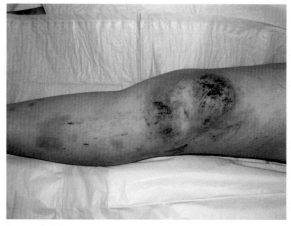

Figure 2-14
Abrasions with red bruising on left knee and shin.

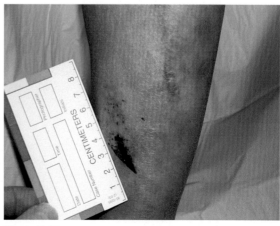

Figure 2-15
Abrasion with red bruising on lower leg.

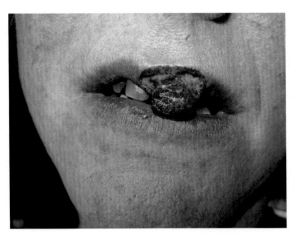

Figure 2-16
Laceration on upper lip.

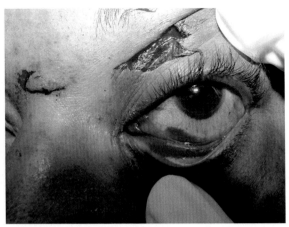

Figure 2-17
Lacerations over the bony surfaces of the glabella and supraorbital ridge; left eye with subconjunctival hemorrhages.

Lacerations may have a variety of wound characteristics depending on the body surface location, depth of laceration, and object used (Figures 2-16 to 2-20). The edges of a laceration are typically irregular or jagged. Abrasions may be present along the wound margins. Bruising may be present in the surrounding tissue. When soft tissue is torn, often there is an incomplete separation of tissue, which results in tissue bridges. With lacerations, the tissue bridges are often small nerves or blood vessels that remain intact and connect the two edges of the wound (Figure 2-21).

Avulsions are caused by the tearing away of a piece of tissue or body part.

This frequently occurs when a force strikes the body at an oblique or tangential angle, and results into the removal of the skin oftentimes extending deep into the underlying fascia or bone (Figure 2-22). Trauma that results in forceful contraction of muscles, ligaments, or tendons can result in avulsion of bones (Eiff, Hatch, Calmbach, 2003).

Skeletal fractures are another form of blunt force trauma.

Fractures are partial or complete breaks in the structure of a bone that occur when more force is applied to the bone than the bone can absorb.

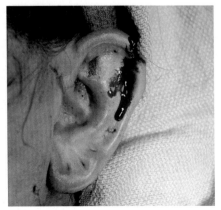

Figure 2-18
Laceration on helix of left pinna.

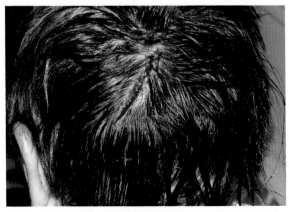

Figure 2-19
Laceration on scalp.

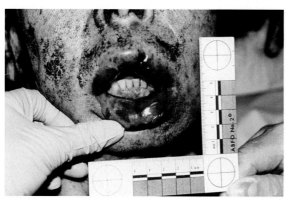

Figure 2-20
Laceration of upper lip with bruising and swelling; bruising and swelling of lower lip also present.

A single incident of trauma like a fall or direct blow, repetitive stress such as running, or pathologic weaknesses in the bone all can result in a fracture. Fractures are classified as open or closed. **Closed fractures**, also called **simple fractures**, refer to bones that are broken

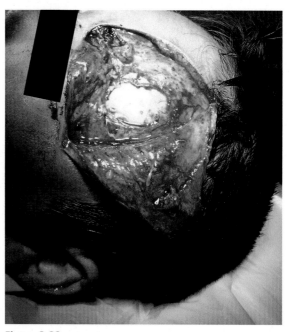

Figure 2-22
Avulsion. Note frontal bone visible.

and the skin remains intact. **Open fractures**, also called **compound fractures**, refer to bones that are broken and exposed due to non-intact skin (Koval, Zuckerman, 2006; Stone, Humphries, 2008; Erkonen, Smith, 2005; Patton, Thibodeau, 2010). Several terms are used to describe fractures based on the type of fracture line, the number of bone fragments, and the force applied to the bone. Common terms for describing fractures include linear, transverse, oblique, spiral, comminuted, segmental, impacted, avulsion, compression, and displaced. Fractures that affect the physis (growth plate) are described using the Salter-Harris classification (Stone, Humphries, 2008; Eiff, Hatch, Calmbach, 2003; Erkonen, Smith, 2005). Although forensic examiners are not typically making the initial diagnosis of skeletal fractures, it is important to understand the mechanisms of skeletal fractures, related terminology, principles of fracture management, and the clinical findings of orthopedic emergencies.

SHARP FORCE TRAUMA

Injures caused by **sharp force trauma** are known as stab or incised wounds (cuts). Sharp force injuries are caused by pointed or edged weapons such as knives.

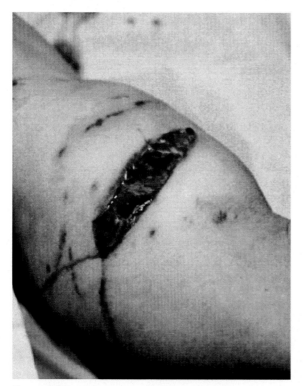

Figure 2-21
Laceration with bridging of tissue on medial aspect of upper arm.

The term laceration should never be used to describe a stab or incised wound.

> A **stab wound** results when a sharp, pointed instrument penetrates the skin and underlying tissue.

Typically, stab wounds are deeper than they are wide; however, this can depend on the type of weapon used. Stab wounds have clearly defined, smooth edges, without tissue bridges, or surrounding abrasions or contusions (Figures 2-23 and 2-24). Although abrasions and contusions are not generally associated with stab wounds, they may be present at the wound edges in the form of a hilt guard pattern. This pattern injury can occur when a knife blade fully penetrates to the hilt with enough force for the hilt guard to subsequently injure the skin upon impact.

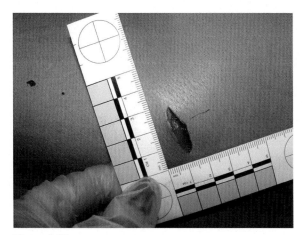

Figure 2-23
  Stab wound.

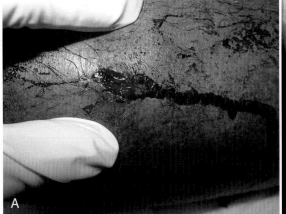

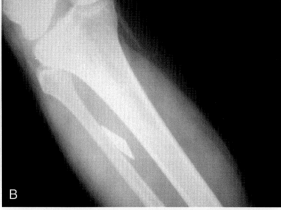

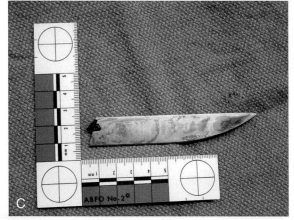

Figure 2-24
  A, Separation of stab wound edges over right tibia. B, X-ray showing knife blade present in soft tissue. C, Knife blade after removal.

An **incised wound** (cut) results when a sharp instrument is dragged along body tissue.

Such wounds are often longer than they are deep. Similar to stab wounds, incised wounds have clearly defined, smooth edges, without tissue bridges, or surrounding abrasions or contusions (Figures 2-25 to 2-27).

PATTERNED INJURIES

Patterned injuries possess characteristics and features indicative of the object or surface that produced them (Olshaker, Olshaker, Smock, 2007) and often can be used to link a particular instrument or object to an injury (Figure 2-28).

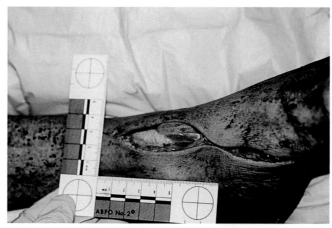

Figure 2-25
Cut on left ankle and foot. Note smooth edges, no tissue bridging.

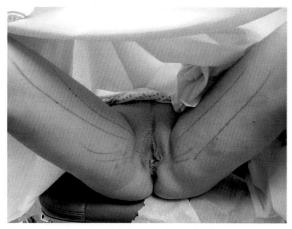

Figure 2-26
Superficial cuts on medial thighs. Note other areas of bruising visible.

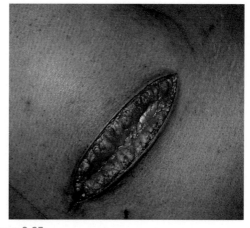

Figure 2-27
Cut on left hip. Note smooth edges, no associated abrasions or bruising and no bridging of tissue.

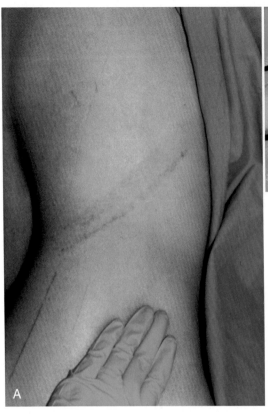

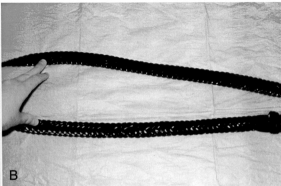

Figure 2-28
A, Patterned bruise on right side of trunk from belt. B, Belt used to inflict patterned bruise in Figure 2-28A.

Common pattern injuries that occur from assaults are finger pad, grip, slap, and drag marks as well as bites and object impressions.

FINGER PAD, GRIP, SLAP, DRAG MARKS

Finger pad marks are 1 to 2-cm circular bruises caused by pressure of the finger pad or tip during grabbing, holding, pressing or squeezing (Figure 2-29). Typically, finger pad bruises are found on the extremities or neck; however, can be found on any body surface area. **Grip marks** refer to a bruise pattern that reflects the grip impression left by the hand. A cluster of finger pad bruises, with three marks (index, middle, ring finger) on one side of the extremity and one mark (thumb) directly opposite, are the most common type of grip marks. Grip marks can also have an elongated bruise pattern that mirrors the length of the entire finger (Figure 2-30). Some grip marks have large

bruises or abrasions on the medial aspect of the upper arm or anterior neck caused by the pressure applied from the palm of the assailant's hand. **Slap marks** can appear as redness with swelling (welts) or bruise patterns that reflect the outline of the palm and fingers as a result of the force of an open hand against the skin (Figure 2-31). **Drag marks** are oval-shaped bruises and abrasions on the skin overlying the spinous processes (Figure 2-32). These are commonly seen as a result of pressure on the bony prominence of the spinous process when the victim is dragged across the floor or ground in the supine position.

BITE MARKS

Human bite marks are frequently present in sexual assault cases. **Bite marks** present in a variety of patterns, which are not always obvious to the forensic examiner. A human bite mark is generally oval or circular in shape and typically comprises two opposing

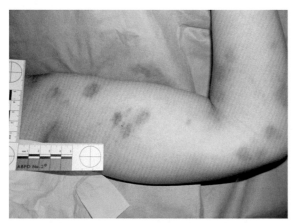

Figure 2-29
Multiple finger pad patterned bruises on left arm.

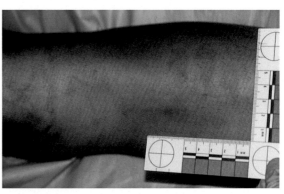

Figure 2-30
Grip mark patterned bruise on left lower leg.

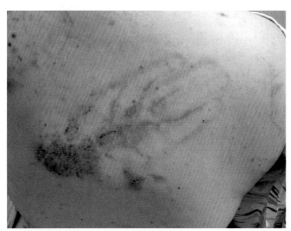

Figure 2-31
Slap mark patterned bruise on back.

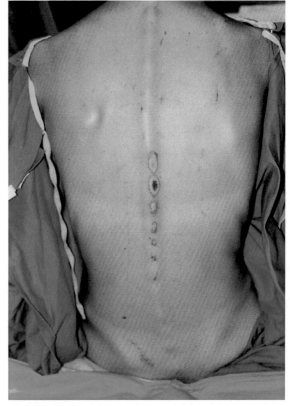

Figure 2-32
Drag mark patterned abrasions over spinous processes.

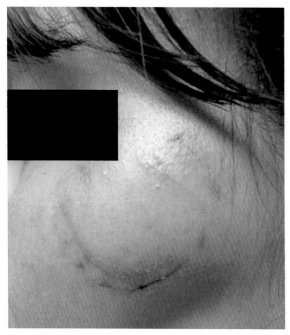

Figure 2-33
Bite mark on left side of face.

U-shaped arches (Figure 2-33). A partial bite mark may have only a single U-shaped arch. Within the arches, there may be individual pattern marks (i.e., bruises, lacerations, abrasions) made by the teeth (Figure 2-34) (Golden, 2011; Hinchliffe, 2011). Central bruising is frequently present as a result of positive or negative pressure in the underlying soft tissue. Central bruising from positive pressure results when the soft tissue is compressed between the teeth during the bite, whereas central bruising from negative pressure results when the soft tissue is pulled into the mouth during suction (Figure 2-35) (Hinchliffe, 2011; Monteleone, Brodeur, 1998). Sometimes this negative pressure bruising is referred to as a "hickey" in lay terms. Bite marks almost always have bruising, but can also have associated swelling, lacerations, and/or abrasions. Document bite marks using accurate, descriptive terms to depict these patterned injuries. Anytime a bite mark is present there is a potential for DNA capture. Saliva is transferred to the skin during the biting process. The examiner should take swabs (per agency or crime lab policy) of the area prior to cleaning or washing the wound. Whenever possible, the forensic examiner should not touch the bite mark without gloves on in order to prevent touch DNA cross contamination.

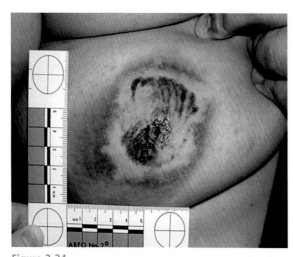

Figure 2-34
Bite mark patterned bruise with teeth marks visible on left breast and nipple.

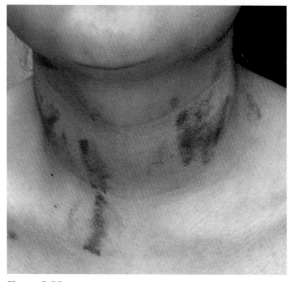

Figure 2-35
Bite mark patterned bruises from suction.

TRAUMATIC ALOPECIA

Traumatic alopecia is the loss of hair as a result of forceful pulling of the scalp hair (Figures 2-36 and 2-37).

In addition to bald areas, bruising may be seen on the scalp from traumatic hair pulling (Figure 2-38). Forensic examiners should carefully inspect the scalp for loose hairs, areas of baldness or bruising, and palpate for areas of tenderness.

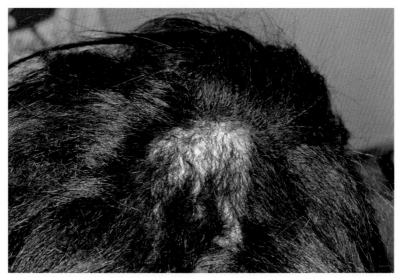
Figure 2-36
Traumatic alopecia on scalp.

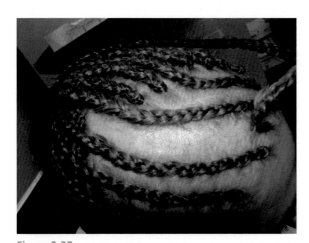
Figure 2-37
Traumatic alopecia on scalp.

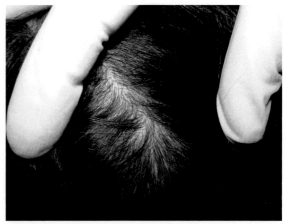
Figure 2-38
Bruising on scalp after hair pulling.

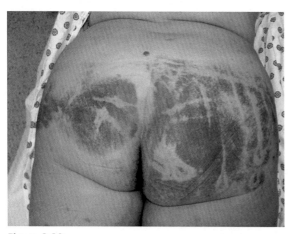

Figure 2-39
  Object patterned bruising on buttocks.

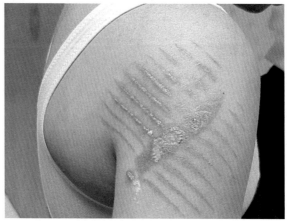

Figure 2-40
  Object patterned wound on right arm and shoulder.

OBJECT PATTERN INJURY

Object pattern injuries demonstrate the outline or impression of the object that caused the wound (Figures 2-39 and 2-40). Usually these are abrasions, bruises, burns, or lacerations. Some of the more common object pattern injuries seen in sexual assaults result from clothing, belts, shoes, jewelry, cords, or rope. Clothing impression pattern bruising on the victim's back can occur when the body weight of the assailant presses the victim's body against a hard surface (Figures 2-41 and 2-42). Impact from being hit, strangled, or tied with a belt, cord, or rope (Figures 2-43 and 2-44), or kicked with shoes or boots (Figure 2-45) can leave pattern impressions on the skin. Necklaces, bracelets, watches, piercings, and rings can all leave pattern impressions if pressed into the skin with enough force.

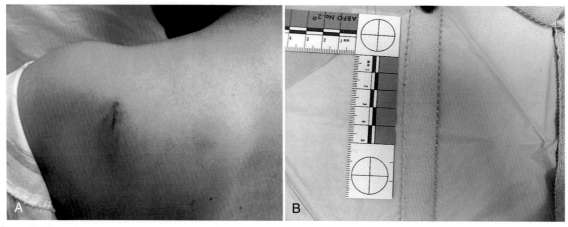

Figure 2-41
  A, Patterned bruise over left scapula from bra strap. B, Bra strap worn at time patterned bruise in Figure 2-41A occurred.

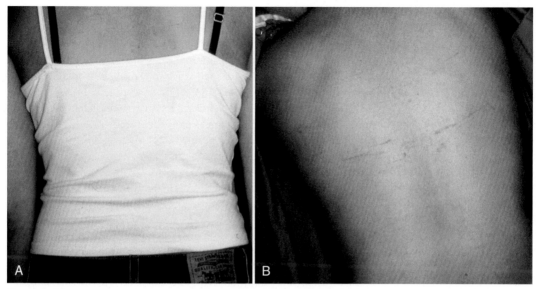

Figure 2-42
A, Shirt and bra worn at time of sexual assault. B, Patterned bruising on back from bra and shirt in Figure 2-42A.

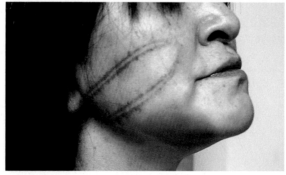

Figure 2-43
Patterned bruise on face from cord.

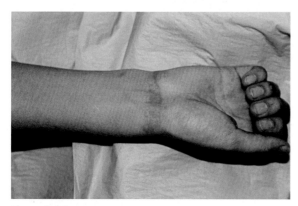

Figure 2-44
Patterned bruising on anterior wrist from rope.

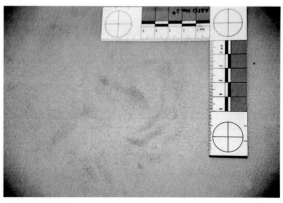

Figure 2-45
Patterned bruise on back after stomped with boot.

DEFENSIVE INJURIES

Injuries that occur on the victim's body from attempts to defend themselves are often referred to as defensive injuries.

Defensive injuries can be in the form of bruises, abrasions, scratches, lacerations, cuts (Figure 2-46), or broken fingernails (Figure 2-47). The injuries occur most commonly on the hands, arms, and legs; however, they can also be found on the victim's back and legs as a result of being curled in a fetal position to protect the head, chest, and abdomen. In strangulation assaults, **defensive injuries** can occur on the victim's neck in the form of fingernail abrasions from the victim's attempt to remove the assailant's hands, arms, legs, or ligature from their neck.

STRANGULATION

Strangulation is a serious, life-threatening form of physical force often used by the assailant during sexual assault.

Strangulation results from external pressure applied to the neck, interrupting oxygen to the brain either by impeding blood flow or respiration. Choking results from an internal obstruction of the airway such as a piece of food stuck in the trachea, or soft tissue swelling from an allergic anaphylactic reaction. Strangulation and choking have two completely different pathophysiologies, and the terms should never be used interchangeably by forensic examiners.

There are numerous signs and symptoms that may occur as a result of a strangulation. Signs of strangulation may include bruising, abrasions, swelling, tenderness, or petechiae (Figures 2-48 to 2-51). Victims may have a single injury, multiple injuries, or no visible external injury after strangulation. Symptoms during strangulation may include difficulty breathing or talking, dizziness, lightheadedness, visual or hearing disturbances, bowel or bladder incontinence, or loss of consciousness. Post-strangulation symptoms may include coughing, vomiting, difficulty breathing, voice changes, sore throat or difficulty swallowing, loss of memory, headache, or neck pain. See Box 2-1 for questions to ask when obtaining a strangulation history from the victim.

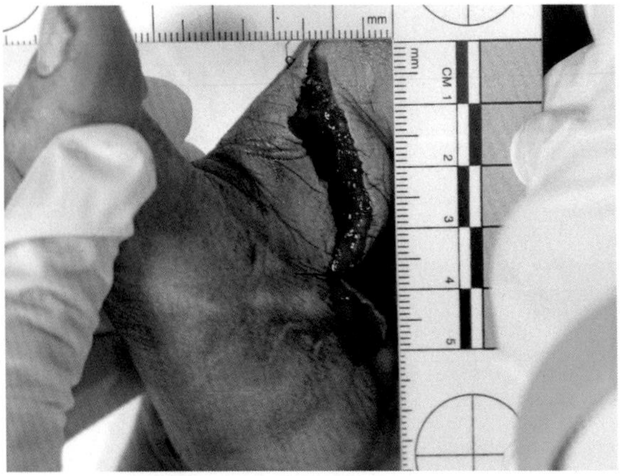

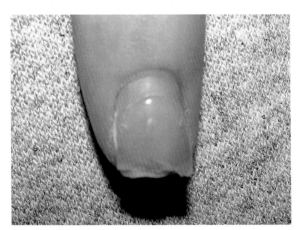

Figure 2-46
Cut on anterior surface of hand; occurred when victim defended self against knife attack.

Figure 2-47
Broken fingernail.

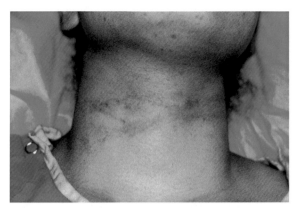

Figure 2-48
Bruising on neck from strangulation.

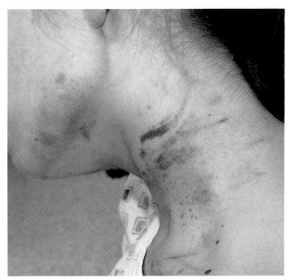

Figure 2-49
Bruising on neck from strangulation.

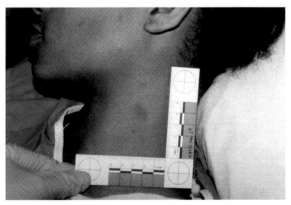

Figure 2-50
Bruising on neck from strangulation; thumb pad patterned bruise.

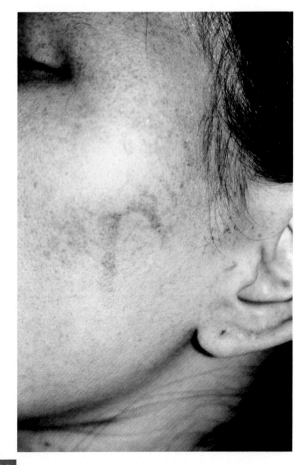

Figure 2-51
Petechiae on face from strangulation. Note patterned bruise on left cheek.

BOX 2-1	Nonfatal Strangulation History Questions

- How was the patient strangled (e.g., one hand, two hand, forearm, ligature)?
- What was the patient's position during strangulation (e.g., sitting, standing, supine, prone)?
- What was the assailant's position in relation to patient during strangulation (e.g., front, back, straddling)?
- How many times did the assailant strangle the patient?
- Approximately how long did each strangulation episode last?
- Was the patient's mouth or nose obstructed (i.e., suffocation)?
- Was the patient's head hit against the wall/floor/ground during strangulation?
- Was the patient's head/neck shaken during the strangulation?
- What did the assailant say to patient during the strangulation?
- What did the patient think was going to happen during the strangulation?
- How did the patient react to the strangulation (e.g., hit, kick, bite, attempt to remove external pressure)?
- What caused the assailant to stop the strangulation (e.g., witness intervened, patient lost consciousness, unknown, etc)?
- Was the strangulation witnessed by children?
- Has the assailant strangled the patient previously (i.e., domestic violence relationship)?
- Did assailant force the patient to have sex?
- Is the patient pregnant?

- Assess for symptoms felt during the strangulation, immediately afterward and currently
  - Did the patient have any breathing changes (e.g., difficulty, unable to breath)?
  - Did the patient have any vision changes (e.g., saw stars, tunnel vision)?
  - Did the patient have any hearing changes (e.g., diminished, muffled)?
  - Did the patient have any voice changes (e.g., difficulty talking, unable to talk)?
  - Did the patient have any swallowing changes (e.g., difficulty swallowing, painful swallowing)?
  - Did the patient have any neurological changes (e.g., dizzy, lightheaded, loss of consciousness)?
  - Did the patient feel any pressure/throbbing in head or eyes?
  - Was the patient incontinent of bladder or bowel?
  - Did the patient have any pain (e.g., neck, head)?
- Assess for signs of strangulation
  - Look for injuries to the head, face, eyes, ears, mouth, neck, shoulders, chest, arms, and hands including bruising, petechiae, swelling, abrasions, lacerations, or point tenderness.

When possible, reexamine patient 24-48 hours after strangulation to reassess for evolving symptoms and signs that may not be present immediately following the assault.

Adapted from "Strangulation Assessment Card," by T. Henry, 2004, *Forensic Nurse Services*.

NON-GENITAL PHYSICAL EXAMINATION

The non-genital physical assessment for the presence or absence of injuries is a major part of any sexual assault examination. Assessment should include the patient's general appearance, obvious odors, active bleeding, deformities, and pain. Pay attention to the patient's body position, posture, and any self-guarding movements. Assessment of the patient's emotional state, behavior, and cognitive abilities should continue throughout the patient encounter. A detailed evaluation of the entire body surface area, using inspection and palpation, should begin at the head and work toward the feet in a systematic fashion, and should be conducted from least invasive to most invasive. Samples of miscellaneous hairs, fibers, debris, or body fluids may need to be collected at the time of the physical assessment to reduce the loss of potential forensic evidence.

Clothing should be assessed for any defects, fluid stains, or debris (Figures 2-52 to 2-55). It is not unusual for clothing items to be missing or present on the body in an abnormal fashion (e.g., inside out, backwards) after a sexual assault (Figure 2-56). Pay close attention to items

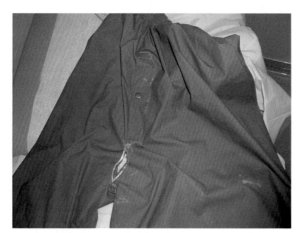

Figure 2-52
Tear in pants.

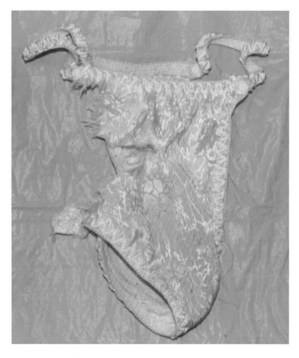

Figure 2-53
Torn underwear.

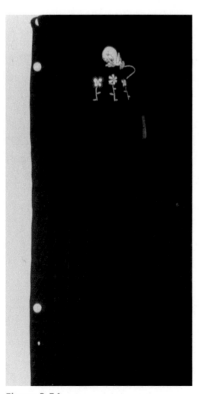

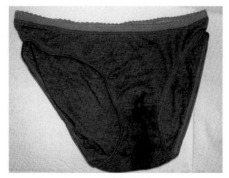

Figure 2-55
Blood on underwear.

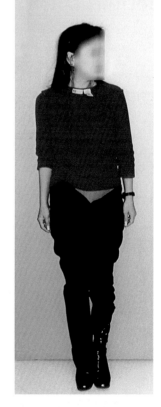

Figure 2-56
Clothing appearance on victim upon arrival to hospital. Note shirt inside out and backwards, pants unbuttoned and unzipped, left pant leg above boot.

Figure 2-54
Buttons missing from shirt.

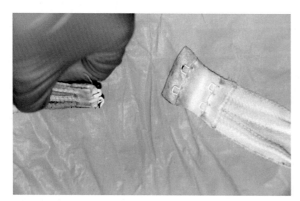

Figure 2-57
Bra hook stretched open.

that can easily be broken such as zippers, snaps, buttons, and bra hooks (Figure 2-57). Assess jewelry for damage or missing parts (Figure 2-58). Skin surfaces should be inspected for any corresponding patterned injuries caused by the clothing or jewelry. Glasses, hearing aids, dentures, or other assistive devices should be assessed for damage (Figures 2-59 and 2-60).

DOCUMENTATION

Comprehensive documentation for sexual assault medical-forensic examinations should include three different types of documentation: narrative, diagrammatic, and photographic.

Narrative documentation is the written narrative of the patient's history of the incident. Throughout the **narrative documentation** of the medical-forensic history, quotation marks should be used to identify exact statements made by the patient. The written narrative should include precise and descriptive details of how any injuries may have occurred, symptoms the patient describes, and post-assault activities that may affect the presence or absence of potential forensic evidence.

Diagrammatic documentation is documentation using drawings of injuries on body maps or diagrams. Diagrammatic documentation of injuries should include location, size, and description. The location of the injury should be drawn on the body part in the correct anatomical location as the actual injury. The size of the injury, measured in centimeters or inches, should be indicated on the diagram. A complete description of the injury should include details such as color, shape, wound margins, presence of debris, bleeding or other body fluids, and tenderness. Any statements made by the patient related to a specific injury should also be noted on the diagram. Each injury on the patient should be documented separately on the body map.

Photographic documentation is documentation using pictures taken by camera of the actual injury. While photographs are a useful form of documentation,

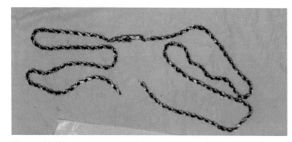

Figure 2-58
Victim's necklace broken during strangulation.

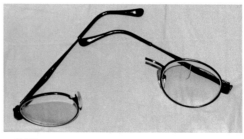

Figure 2-59
Victim's eyeglasses broken when punched in face.

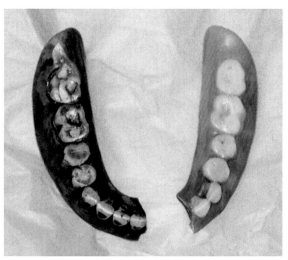

Figure 2-60
Victim's dentures broken when punched in face; left side of denture fell
out of mouth during assault, right side of denture remained in place.

they should never be the only form of documentation used. Photographic documentation is done in conjunction with narrative and diagrammatic documentation; never in place of. Initial documentation of injury on the body maps should be done at the time of the examination, not from a photograph at a later date.

Medical photography is used in many specialties to document physical assessments or procedures. For sexual assault examinations, medical photography has several purposes. Combined with narrative and diagrammatic documentation, medical photography provides a thorough medical record of the episode of care provided. It enables the examiner to consult with other medical professionals regarding the physical findings if needed, and it allows for peer review and quality assurance review. Access to consultation, peer review, and quality assurance reviews are critical to the improvement of patient care. If sexual assault criminal charges are filed, agencies within the criminal justice system may choose to subpoena the medical records and use the photographic documentation as evidence in the prosecution and defense of the crime.

> Written consent must be obtained from the patient in order to photograph their body.

It is critical that the principles of informed consent are followed as part of the consent process. The necessity and purpose of the photographs as well as who has legal access to the photographs should be discussed in detail. As part of the informed consent process, the patient should be provided the opportunity to ask questions prior to consenting or declining the photographing of their body. An additional, separate, written consent must be obtained from the patient in order for the examiner to release copies of the photographs to law enforcement. If written consent is not obtained from the patient, the photographs can only be released with a court order.

> Photographs taken during a medical-forensic examination are part of the medical record.

Agencies must have a policy in place regarding how to manage photographs and digital images, how images are released to law enforcement, and how photographs will be stored with the medical record.

> Management of photographic medical records must comply with federal and state healthcare laws.

See Box 2-2 for specific applicable federal regulations.

| **BOX 2-2** | **Healthcare Regulations Pertaining to Electronic Health Records and Digital Photographs** |

HEALTH INSURANCE PORTABILITY AND ACCOUNTABILITY ACT (HIPAA)
- 45 CFR 164.308(a)(1) – Administrative Safeguards - Security Management Process
- 45 CFR 164.308(a)(6) – Administrative Safeguards - Security Incident Procedures
- 45 CFR 164.310(d)(1) – Physical Safeguards -Media and Device Control
- 45 CFR 164.312(a) – Technical Safeguards - Access Control
- 45 CFR 164.312(b) – Technical Safeguards -Audit Controls
- 45 CFR 164.312(e)(1) – Technical Safeguards -Transmission Security
- 45 CFR 164.404, .406, and .408 - Data Breach Notification to Individuals
- 45 CFR 164.406 Data Breach Notification to the Media
- 45 CFR 164.408 Data Breach Notification to the Secretary
- 45 CFR 170.302(r) General Certification Criteria – Audit Log

HEALTH INFORMATION TECHNOLOGY FOR ECONOMIC AND CLINICAL HEALTH (HITECH) ACT
- Widens scope of privacy and security protections available under HIPAA
- Increases legal liability for noncompliance
- Provides for enhanced enforcement of HIPAA compliance

From Electronic Code of Federal Regulations (n.d.). Retrieved June 9, 2011, from GPO Access http://ecfr.gpoaccess.gov/cgi/t/text/text-idx?c=ecfr&tpl=%2Findex.tpl
Health Information Technology for Economic and Clinical Health Act. (2009). Retrieved June 9, 2011, from HIPAA Survival Guide website: http://www.hipaasurvivalguide.com/hitech-act-text.php

NON-GENITAL PHOTOGRAPHY

Digital cameras are currently the most widely used and accepted technology for photographing injuries. Rarely are Polaroid or 35mm film cameras used for this purpose in the United States today. Policies should be established that cover photography protocols, informed consent, storage of photographs in the medical record, and release of photographs. Healthcare agencies should be familiar and compliant with security regulations that pertain to electronic health records, including photographs (see Box 2-2).

The examiner should establish a routine for photographing injuries. One routine that ensures consistency in the documentation of identified injuries, is to take photographs at the same time as diagramming them on body maps during the physical assessment. It is recommended that the examiner start the photography process by taking identification photographs first. Begin with a photograph of a patient label that includes the patient's name, date of birth, medical record number, date of exam, and examining nurse's name. Next, take an overall photograph of the clothed patient. This can serve as an identification photograph, as well as document the patient's general appearance at the time of the examination.

Photographing injuries should follow three main principles (often referred to as the Rule of Three). First, take an orientation photograph of the injured area to show its location on the body surface in relation to anatomical landmarks on the body. Second, take a medium range image of the injury. Third, take two close-up images of the injury for detail; one image using an appropriate ruler or scale, and one image without. Photographs should be free of distortion and be an accurate representation of the injury visualized by the examiner in person. When possible, the photographs should be free of distractors (e.g., other people in room, plants, equipment, paperwork). Every effort should be made by the examiner to minimize the patient's discomfort by maintaining the patient's privacy and modesty. Careful positioning of the patient and the use of drapes or sheets can minimize unnecessary exposure of other body surfaces while taking photographs of the injury.

Wound identification and documentation is an integral component of medical-forensic examinations of patients who have suffered physical and sexual assaults. It is imperative for forensic examiners to be knowledgeable in anatomy, physiology, mechanisms of injury, wound assessment, and documentation methods. Research pertaining to wound pathophysiology continues to evolve; therefore, forensic examiners must ensure they remain abreast of the science to maintain current evidence-based practices.

Key Terms

Abrasion
Avulsion
Bilirubin
Biliverdin
Bite mark
Blunt force trauma
Bruise
Closed fracture
Compound fracture
Contusion
Cut
Defensive injury
Diagrammatic documentation
Drag mark
Ecchymosis
Erythrocyte
Finger pad mark
Fracture
Grip mark
Hemoglobin
Incised wound
Laceration
Macrophage
Narrative documentation
Object pattern injury
Open fracture
Patterned injury
Petechiae
Photographic documentation
Sharp force trauma
Simple fracture
Slap mark
Stab wound
Strangulation
Traumatic alopecia

References

Besant-Matthews, P. (2011). Blunt, sharp, and firearm injuries. In V. Lynch, & J. Duval (Eds.), *Forensic Nursing Science* (2nd ed.). St. Louis, MO: Elsevier Mosby.

Di Maio, D. J., & Di Maio, V. J. (2001). *Forensic pathology* (2nd ed.). Boca Raton, FL: CRC Press.

Eiff, M., Hatch, R., & Calmbach, W. (2003). *Fracture management for primary care.* Philadelphia: Saunders.

Erkonen, W., & Smith, W. (2005). *Radiology 101: The basics and fundamentals of imaging* (2nd ed.). Philadelphia: Lippincott, Williams & Wilkins.

Golden, G. (2011). Bite mark injuries. In V. Lynch, & J. Duval (eds.), *Forensic Nursing Science* (2nd ed.). St. Louis, MO: Elsevier Mosby.

Hinchliffe, J. (2011). Forensic odontology, part 4. Human bite marks. *British Dental Journal, 210* (8), 363–368.

Hughes, V., Ellis, P., Burt, T., & Langlois, N. (2004). The practical application of reflectance spectrophotometry for the demonstration of haemoglobin and its degradation in bruises. *Journal of Clinical Pathology, 57* (4), 355–359.

Hughes, V., Ellis, P., & Langlois, N. (2004). The perception of yellow in bruises. *Journal of Clinical Forensic Medicine, 11* (5), 257–259.

Koval, K., & Zuckerman, J. (2006). *Handbook of fractures* (3rd ed.). Philadelphia: Lippincott, Williams & Wilkins.

Langlois, N. (2007). The science behind the quest to determine the age of bruises—a review of the English language literature. *Forensic Science, Medicine, and Pathology, 3* (4), 241–251.

Monteleone, J., & Brodeur, A. (1998). *Child maltreatment: A clinical guide and reference* (2nd ed.). St. Louis, MO: G.W. Medical Publishing, Inc.

Nash, K., & Sheridan, D. (2009). Can one accurately date a bruise? State of the science. *Journal of Forensic Nursing, 5* (1), 31–37.

Olshaker, J., Olshaker, M., & Smock, W. (2007). *Forensic emergency medicine* (2nd ed.). Philadelphia: Lippincott, Williams & Wilkins.

Patton, K., & Thibodeau, G. (2010). *Anatomy and physiology* (7th ed.). St. Louis, MO: Elsevier.

Spitz, W. (2006). *Spitz and Fisher's medicolegal investigation of death* (4th ed.). Springfield, IL: Thomas.

Stone, C., & Humphries, R. (2008). *CURRENT diagnosis and treatment emergency medicine* (6th ed.). New York: McGraw-Hill.

Yajima, Y., & Funayama, M. (2006). Spectrophotometric and tristimulus analysis of the colors of subcutaneous bleeding in living persons. *Forensic Science International, 156* (2–3), 131–137.

CHAPTER 3

ANATOMY AND PHYSIOLOGY

Kimberly Wieczorek

ADULT AND ADOLESCENT ANATOMY AND PHYSIOLOGY

Understanding normal anatomy and physiology in adults and adolescents forms the foundation for the identification and interpretation of findings associated with a sexual assault. Fundamental knowledge regarding oral, genital, and anorectal anatomy and physiology should include an in-depth understanding of normal anatomy and physiology, normal anatomical variants, and developmental changes across the lifespan.

FEMALE GENITAL ANATOMY
External Genitalia

There are two collective terms used to describe the female **external genitalia,** the vulva and the vestibule. The **vulva** includes the mons pubis, labia majora, labia minora, clitoris, vestibule, and perineum (Figure 3-1). The **vestibule** is bordered by the clitoris, inner aspects of the labia minora and the posterior fourchette and includes the urethral os, hymen, **vaginal introitus,** Bartholin and Skene glands and the fossa navicularis (Figure 3-2) (Lawton, Littlewood, 2006; Puppo, 2011). Because the terms vulva and vestibule represent multiple collective structures, their use for identifying the location of findings, trauma, or evidence should be limited in order to avoid confusion regarding the

actual structure(s) involved. For example, documenting that a patient has a linear break in the skin integrity to the vulva does not indicate whether the finding is located on the mons pubis, labia majora, labia minora, clitoris or perineum.

The female external genitalia include the mons pubis, labia majora, labia minora, anterior commissure, clitoris, urethral os, posterior fourchette, fossa navicularis, perineum, Bartholin glands, Skene glands, hymen and the vaginal introitus (Figure 3-3).

The **mons pubis,** which forms the anterior boundary of the female genitalia and covers the **symphysis pubis,** is composed primarily of adipose or fat tissue covered by keratinized, stratified squamous epithelium. Hormonal influences associated with puberty result in the growth of coarse pubic hair over the mons pubis, which extends posteriorly to the outer aspect of the labia majora (Bikoo, 2007; Farage, Maibach, 2006).

The **labia majora,** or outer larger lips, form the lateral boundaries of the female genitalia and are primarily composed of **adipose tissue** covered by a thin layer of smooth muscle and keratinized, stratified squamous epithelial tissue (Farage, Maibach, 2006). The size of the labia majora are impacted by an individual's overall body mass. Females with excessive adipose tissue may have enlarged labia majora, whereas females who are underweight may have less

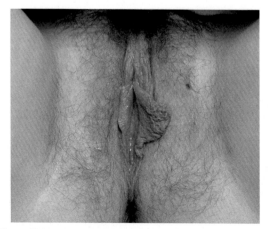

Figure 3-1
The vulva is composed of the mons pubis, labia majora, labia minora, clitoris and perineum.

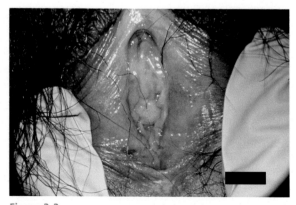

Figure 3-2
The vestibule is bordered by the clitoris, inner aspects of the labia minora and the posterior fourchette and includes the urethral os, hymen, vaginal introitus, Bartholin glands, Skene glands, and the fossa navicularis.

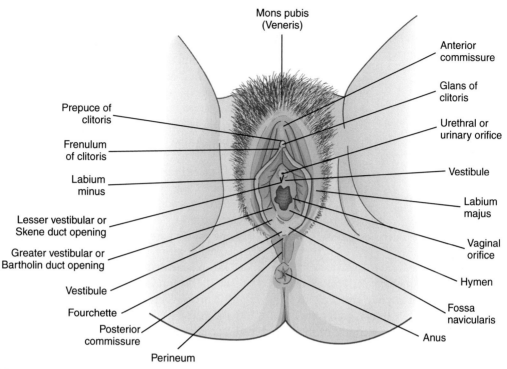

Mons pubis
(Veneris)

Anterior
commissure

Glans of
clitoris

Prepuce of
clitoris

Urethral or
urinary orifice

Frenulum
of clitoris

Vestibule

Labium
minus

Labium
majus

Lesser vestibular or
Skene duct opening

Greater vestibular or
Bartholin duct opening

Vaginal
orifice

Vestibule

Hymen

Fourchette

Fossa
navicularis

Posterior
commissure

Anus

Perineum

Figure 3-3
Female external genitalia. (From McCance, K. L. (2010). *Pathophysiology: The biologic basis for disease in adults and children.* (6th ed.). St. Louis, MO: Mosby.

pronounced labia majora. In addition, asymmetrical labia majora are not uncommon, with one labium majus being larger or more prominent than the other (see Figure 3-1). There are numerous **sudoriferous** (sweat) and **sebaceous** (oil) **glands** and hair follicles located within the labia majora. Pubic hair may fully cover

the outer aspects of the labia majora or be sparse as depicted in Figure 3-4. The labia majora may become inflamed, irritated, or clogged during puberty or with shaving (Figure 3-5), which has become more common in adolescent and adult females (Berek, Novak, 2007; Bikoo, 2007; Lawton, Littlewood, 2006).

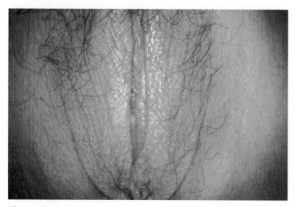

Figure 3-4
Labia majora; postpubertal female.

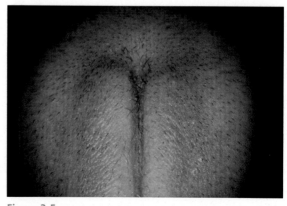

Figure 3-5
Folliculitis associated with shaving; labia majora; postpubertal female.

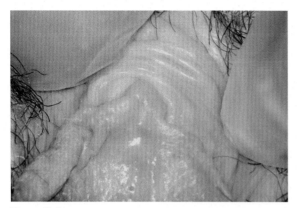

Figure 3-6
Manual retraction of the anterior commissure or clitoral hood allows for visualization of clitoris; postpubertal female.

The **labia minora,** or inner smaller lips, are located between the labia majora and unite anteriorly to form the anterior commissure or prepuce in both prepubertal and postpubertal women and posteriorly to form the posterior fourchette in postpubertal females. The labia minora are hairless folds of connective tissue covered by keratinized, stratified squamous epithelium with numerous sebaceous glands and an abundant vascular network (Farage, Maibach, 2006). This vascular network is responsible for the labia minora appearing red in color in postpubertal females (Berek, Novak, 2007). As with the labia majora, the labia minora may be asymmetrical in appearance (Lawton, Littlewood, 2006; Puppo, 2011; Yang, Cold, Yilmaz, Maravilla, 2005).

The **anterior commissure** created by the labia minora forms the clitoral hood or prepuce, which covers the **clitoris** anteriorly (Figure 3-6). The clitoral hood is composed of keratinized, stratified squamous epithelium (Farage, Maibach, 2006). The female clitoris, which is approximately 2 to 3 cm in length, is analogous to the male penis. The clitoris is composed of two columns of erectile tissue, which become engorged during sexual arousal (Puppo, 2011; Yang, Cold, Yilmaz, Maravilla, 2005).

The urethral os or opening is located below the clitoris (Yang, Cold, Yilmaz, Maravilla, 2005). The urethral os is bordered by two Skene glands at approximately the 11 o'clock and the 1 o'clock positions. The **Skene glands** are rarely seen or felt unless they become inflamed or infected (Berek, Novak, 2007).

The **posterior fourchette** is a band or bridge of tissue that is formed by the union of the labia minora posteriorly (Figure 3-7). This area is often referred to as the posterior commissure in prepubertal females. The posterior fourchette or commissure is a relatively weak anatomical structure. As a result, injury to the posterior fourchette during sexual activity, tampon insertion, or anogenital inspections using labial separation, labial traction, or speculum insertion are not uncommon (Lawton, Littlewood, 2006).

As shown in Figure 3-8, the **fossa navicularis** is a slightly concave depressed area located inferiorly to the hymen and anteriorly to the posterior fourchette (Ostrzenski, 2002). The **Bartholin glands** are located lateral to the fossa navicularis within the inner aspects

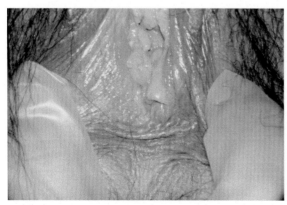

Figure 3-7
Posterior fourchette visualized using labial separation.

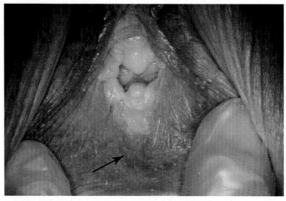

Figure 3-8
Concave depression known as the fossa navicularis.

of the labia minora at approximately the 5 o'clock and the 7 o'clock positions (Berek, Novak, 2007). The Bartholin glands secrete fluid that assists with vaginal lubrication during sexual intercourse (Perry-Philo, Bradford, 2007). As with the Skene glands, the Bartholin glands are rarely seen or palpated unless inflamed or irritated.

The **hymen** is a thin, non-keratinized membrane that surrounds or partially covers the vaginal introitus (Farage, Maibach, 2006). All female children, in the absence of rare congenital abnormalities, are born with a hymen (Hobday, Haury, Dayton, 1997; McCann, Wells, Simon, Voris, 1990). Hymenal configurations vary and include crescentic, annular, septate, imperforate, cribiform, and fimbriated (McCann, Wells, Simon, Voris, 1990). Studies have shown that the majority of children are born with an annular hymen, which progresses to a crescentic shape as maternal estrogen levels decrease (Berenson, 1995). A **crescentic hymen** has anterior attachments in the anterior portion of the hymen between the 9 o'clock and the 3 o'clock positions, with the most common at approximately the 11 o'clock and the 1 o'clock positions. Between these two attachment points, there is an absence of hymenal tissue (see Figure 3-26). This absence of hymenal tissue should not be mistaken for healed hymenal trauma. An **annular hymen** extends circumferentially around the vaginal introitus as shown in Figure 3-9. A **septate hymen** has one or more bands of hymenal tissue that cross the vaginal

introitus creating multiple openings (Heger, Ticson, Guerra, et al., 2002). Remnants of septate hymenal tissue are often seen in adolescents and adults after estrogenization and sexual intercourse as demonstrated by the hymenal tags at the 12 o'clock and the 5 o'clock positions in Figure 3-10. An **imperforate hymen** completely covers the vaginal introitus and results from congenital failure of the inferior end of the vagina to perforate the hymen during the perinatal period of development (Nucci, Oliva, 2009). Having the patient bear down may help differentiate between an imperforate hymen and vaginal agenesis. Bearing down as if to have a bowel movement typically causes an imperforate hymen to bulge outward, whereas it will have no effect on the appearance of the genitalia of a female with vaginal agenesis. Imperforate hymens not identified or corrected prior to the onset of puberty and menses may result in the collection of blood in the vaginal vault, thereby requiring surgical intervention (Nucci, Oliva, 2009). A **cribiform hymen** has multiple, irregularly sized openings and a microperforate hymen has a smaller diameter opening. A **fimbriated** or redundant hymen is frequently seen in postpubertal women as a result of estrogenization and is characterized by multiple scalloped projections along the hymenal rim and rolled edges (Heger, Ticson, Guerra, et al., 2002; Myhre, Myklestad, Adams, 2010).

The **perineum,** which forms the posterior boundary of the external genitalia, extends from the posterior

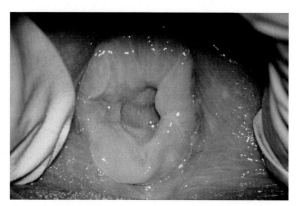

Figure 3-9
Fully estrogenized, annular hymen.

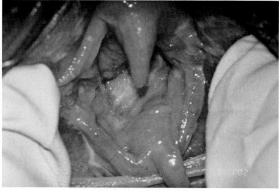

Figure 3-10
Septate hymenal remnants at the 12 o'clock & the 5 o'clock positions.

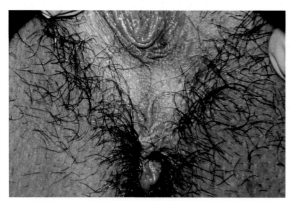

Figure 3-11
Female perineum extending from the posterior fourchette to the perianal folds.

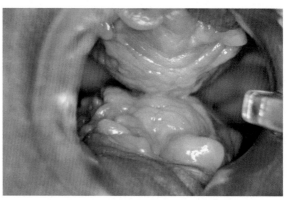

Figure 3-12
Anterior and posterior vaginal columns visualized with speculum insertion.

fourchette or commissure to the anus in females (Figure 3-11) and from the base of the scrotum to the anus in males. The perineum is composed of keratinized, stratified squamous epithelium (Farage, Maibach, 2006). The perineal body located underneath the perineal skin is the point of union of the perineal muscles and is responsible for forming the support structures of the pelvic floor (Berek, Novak, 2007; Lawton, Littlewood, 2006).

Internal Genitalia

The **vagina** is a distensible tube lined with non-keratinized, fibromuscular tissue that extends from the vestibule to the cervix (Bikoo, 2007; Farage, Maibach, 2006; Yang, Cold, Yilmaz, Maravilla, 2005). The **vaginal**

columns (longitudinal ridges) extend the length of the anterior and posterior vaginal walls (Figures 3-12 and 3-13), while the **vaginal rugae (transverse folds)** are found laterally as shown in Figures 3-14 and 3-15 (Berenson, 1998). The anterior vaginal column may extend downward into the vaginal vault in women with **cystoceles** (Figure 3-16) and the posterior vaginal column may protrude upward into the vagina with a **rectocele** (Figure 3-17). The intravaginal **longitudinal ridges** frequently attach to or overlap the posterior aspect of the hymen resulting in hymenal mounds (Heger, Ticson, Guerra, et al., 2002). The posterior vaginal wall is approximately 3 cm longer than the anterior vaginal wall. The spaces created by the attachment of the vagina to the cervix are referred to as the

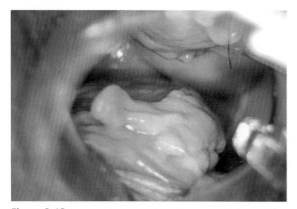

Figure 3-13
Anterior and posterior vaginal columns visualized with speculum insertion.

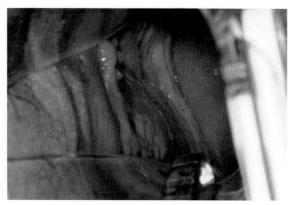

Figure 3-14
Vaginal rugae visualized with speculum insertion.

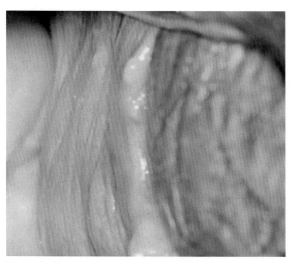

Figure 3-15
Vaginal rugae visualized with speculum insertion.

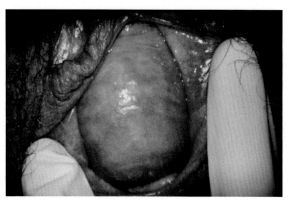

Figure 3-16
Cystocele.

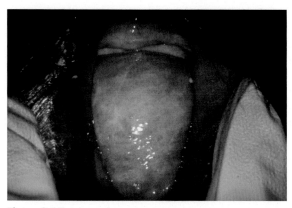

Figure 3-17
Rectocele.

anterior, posterior and lateral fornices (Berek, Novak, 2007). Vaginal lubrication is produced by engorgement of the vasculature surrounding the vagina and subsequent transudate production. In prepubertal and postmenopausal females, the vaginal epithelium is relatively thin and atrophic (Figures 3-18 and 3-19) with a neutral pH. In contrast, in pubertal females, the presence of endogenous estrogen results in thickening of the vaginal epithelium and the growth of lactobacilli, which acidifies the vaginal pH. The difference in vaginal pH when comparing prepubertal and **postmenopausal** females to pubertal females is important in regard to the characteristics of bacterial colonization in each age range. Bacterial colonization in prepubertal and

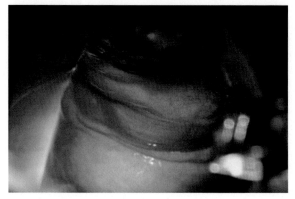

Figure 3-18
Atrophic anterior vaginal wall of a postmenopausal female. Note the decreased rugae.

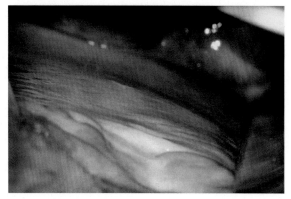

Figure 3-19
Atrophic posterior vaginal wall of a postmenopausal female. Note the decreased rugae.

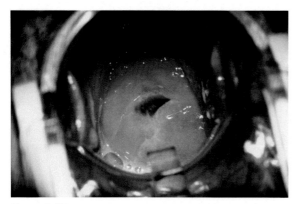

Figure 3-20
Cervix without ectropion tissue visible.

postmenopausal females is often enteric in nature, whereas the acidic environment associated with puberty prevents such colonization (Farage, Maibach, 2006; Kelley, 2007). In addition, the relatively neutral vaginal pH found in prepubertal females necessitates the use of alternative sexually transmitted disease culture media in order to avoid erroneous false positives associated with rapid assay testing.

The **cervix** is the distal most portion of the uterus as shown in Figure 3-20 (Berek, Novak, 2007). The surface of the cervix is covered by stratified squamous epithelium except during the newborn period, puberty, and childbearing years and with the use of birth control pills or estrogen replacement therapy. During these periods of time, the columnar epithelium, which is usually located in the endocervical canal extends out onto the face of the cervix creating a rough, red, and sometimes irregular area (Figures 3-21 and 3-22). This area is referred to as ectropion tissue and should not be misinterpreted for trauma associated with an assault or a disease process. The area where the stratified squamous epithelium and columnar epithelium merge is referred to as the squamocolumnar junction or the transformation zone (Berek, Novak, 2007; Matiluko, 2009) and is the site for many precancerous and cancerous cervical lesions.

The **uterus** is composed of three layers, the endometrium or inner layer, the myometrium or middle layer, and the perimetrium or outermost layer. In postpubertal women, the endometrial layer sheds approximately every 28 days during menses in response to hormonal changes. During a normal pregnancy, the fertilized egg implants in the endometrium where it stays for the remainder of the pregnancy. The myometrium is composed of smooth muscle and is responsible for the muscular contractions necessary to move the fetus into the birth canal during delivery (Marieb, 2006; Perry-Philo, Bradford, 2007).

The ovaries are analogous to the male testes and are responsible for the production of ova or eggs and both estrogen and progesterone. Ova are released into the fallopian tubes, which serve as the site for fertilization. Parastaltic waves move the fertilized ova through the fallopian tubes into the uterus where implantation occurs in a normal pregnancy (Marieb, 2006; Perry-Philo, Bradford, 2007).

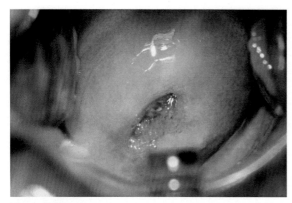

Figure 3-21
Ectropion tissue at the cervical os of postpubertal female. Area where the columnar epithelium meets the squamous epithelium is referred to as the transformation zone.

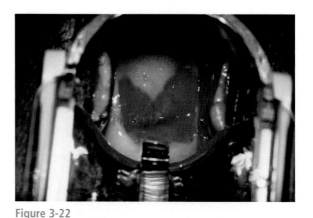

Figure 3-22
Extensive cervical ectropion tissue. The amount of ectropion tissue various among individuals and may be minimal, extensive, or appear in patches that are dispersed across the face of the cervix.

MALE GENITAL ANATOMY AND PHYSIOLOGY

Unlike females, most of the male reproductive system is located outside of the body. The male external genitalia include the penis, scrotum, and testicles. The internal genitalia include accessory organs, the ducts, and glands. Figure 3-23 identifies the male external and internal genitalia.

External Genitalia

The **penis** is covered with keratinized tissue externally and structurally includes the shaft, glans, and prepuce. The **penile shaft** extends from the **foreskin** to the pubis and is composed of three cylindrical compartments, namely two **corpora cavernosa** and the **corpus spongiosum,** which consist of erectile tissue and a vascular network (Ceo, 2006; Kochhar, Taylor, Sangar, 2010). The **urethra** runs through the corpus spongiosum. The **glans** is the distal end of the penis and contains the urethral opening. The **prepuce** or foreskin covers the glans (Figure 3-24). The foreskin is surgically removed during circumcision (see Figure 3-25) (Ceo, 2006; Marieb, 2006).

The **scrotum** is a protective sac composed of two compartments that contain the testes. The scrotal skin is thin, has rugae, contains sebaceous glands, and is sparsely covered with pubic hair (see Figure 3-24). Connective tissue and smooth muscle underlying the skin cause the scrotum to appear wrinkled and help to maintain an adequate environmental temperature for the testes and sperm production (Ceo, 2006; Perry-Philo, Bradford, 2007).

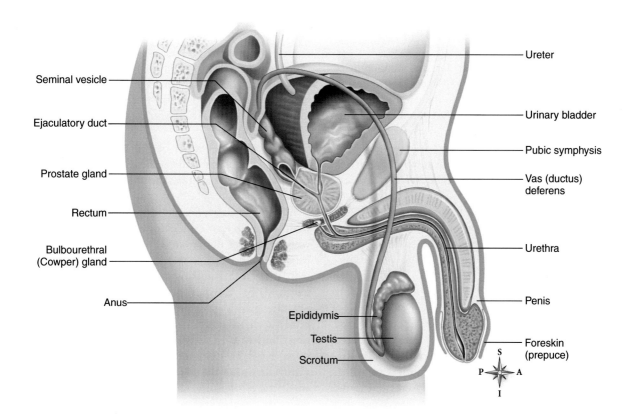

Figure 3-23

Male reproductive anatomy. (From Patton K. T. , & Thibodeau G. A. (2010). *Anatomy & physiology.* (7th ed.). St Louis, MO: Mosby.)

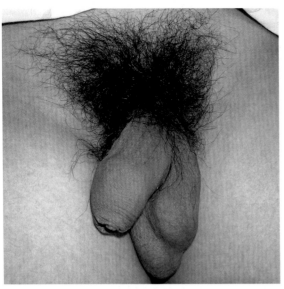

Figure 3-24
Male external genitalia. Uncircumcised prepuce covers the glans.

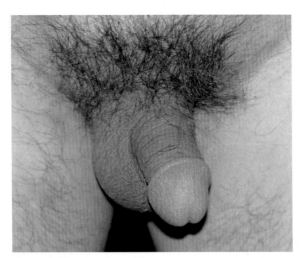

Figure 3-25
Male external genitalia, circumsized.

The **testes** are responsible for the production of **sperm** and **testosterone.** Each testis is enclosed in fibrous, connective tissue and contains the **epididymis** and **seminiferous tubules.** Sperm are produced in the seminiferous tubules and then transported to the epididymis for temporary storage. It takes approximately twenty days for sperm to move through the epididymis, during which time the sperm mature (Ceo, 2006; Perry-Philo, Bradford, 2007). Once mature, sperm are composed of a head, a tail, and a midpiece (Ostrzenski, 2002). During sexual stimulation, the epididymis contracts propelling the sperm into the vas deferens (Ceo, 2006; Marieb, 2006; Perry-Philo, Bradford, 2007).

INTERNAL GENITALIA

The **vas deferens** is encased in the spermatic cord along with blood vessels and nerves. A spermatic cord attaches to each testis, overlaps the bladder in the pelvic cavity, and ends in the ejaculatory duct, which empties into the urethra. The primary function of the vas deferens is to move mature sperm into the urethra during ejaculation. The vas deferens is cauterized or incised during a vasectomy. The urethra, the terminal point of the male reproductive duct system, functions to transport both urine and sperm. During ejaculation,

the internal urethra sphincter closes as sperm enters the urethra, thereby preventing urine from mixing with the ejaculate and sperm from entering the urinary bladder (Ceo, 2006; Marieb, 2006; Perry-Philo, Bradford, 2007).

The **accessory glands** of the male reproductive tract include the seminal vesicles, prostate gland and the bulbourethral glands. The seminal vesicles produce approximately 60% of seminal fluid, a glucose rich fluid, which is released into the ejaculatory duct with sperm during ejaculation. The **prostate gland,** which encircles the proximal portion of the urethra, produces fluid that is released from several ducts into the urethra during ejaculation. The **bulbourethral** or **Cowper glands,** located below the prostate gland, produce mucus, which is released into the distal urethra prior to ejaculation. Sperm function less effectively in an acidic environment. It is believed the fluid secreted by the bulbourethral glands may alter the pH of the urethra by removing small traces of urine, thereby creating an environment that maximizes sperm motility and viability. With each **ejaculation,** approximately 2 to 5 mL of seminal fluid are released from the accessory glands containing approximately 50 to 130 million sperm per mL (Marieb, 2006; Perry-Philo, Bradford, 2007).

CHANGES ASSOCIATED WITH PUBERTY

The onset of **puberty** reflects reproductive development in both males and females. Changes associated with puberty in North American females occurs between the ages of eight and thirteen and in males between the ages of nine and fourteen. At the onset of puberty, the initial external signs in females are breast budding and pubic hair growth and in males are penile and scrotal elongation and pubic hair growth. Secondary sexual characteristics in females may develop as early as five years before the onset of menses. The average age of menarche in females is between 12 and 13 years of age (Farage, Maibach, 2006).

ESTROGENIZATION

The presence or absence of **estrogen** impacts the appearance of the female genitalia across the lifespan (Farage, Maibach, 2006; Kelley, 2007). At birth up until approximately four weeks of age, the appearance of a newborn female's genitalia is directly affected by maternal estrogen transmitted through the placenta prior to birth. During this period of time, a newborn's genitalia may be edematous with vaginal discharge similar to that seen in postpubertal females. Newborns may experience vaginal bleeding shortly after birth before maternal estrogen levels decrease (Farage, Maibach, 2006).

Changes in hymenal and vulvar-vestibular tissue in prepubertal females have not been systematically studied. However, anecdotal evidence reveals that there is variability among individual girl's genital appearance from approximately three to six years of age until changes associated with puberty begin to occur. During this period of time, in response to a decrease in endogenous estrogen levels, the genital tissue is relatively **atrophic** in most females (Farage, Maibach, 2006). The genitalia may appear red during the prepubertal period because the tissue is thinner and the vasculature is therefore closer to the surface (Figure 3-26). In prepubertal females, the hymen is thin to translucent as indicated in Figure 3-27 and painful to touch (Berenson, 1995). The vaginal pH is basic (Farage, Maibach, 2006) and if the cervix is visualized, ectropion tissue will be absent. The administration of exogenous estrogen will change the appearance of the hymen at this developmental stage causing changes similar to those associated with the onset of puberty.

As a female progresses toward puberty, endogenous estrogen levels begin to increase until reaching peak levels during childbearing years and pregnancy. As estrogen levels increase, the vaginal epithelium thicken, vaginal secretions increase, and the vaginal pH changes from relatively neutral to acidic. Leukorrhea associated with puberty results from the desquamation of epithelial cells in response to increasing estrogen. The labia majora, labia minora, and clitoris enlarge and the vestibular glands begin secreting fluid (Farage, Maibach,

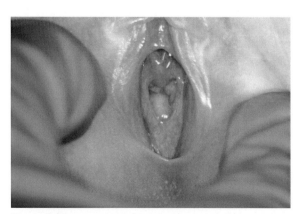

Figure 3-26
 Normal, thin, vascular, translucent, non-estrogenized, crescentic hymen; prepubertal female.

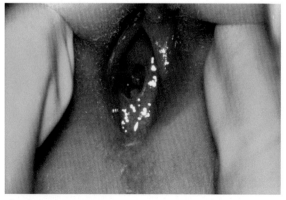

Figure 3-27
 Non-estrogenized, crescentic hymen; prepubertal female. Note the normal hymenal redness caused by the pronounced vasculature associated with non-estrogenized genital tissue.

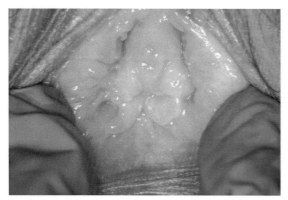

Figure 3-28
Fully estrogenized, redundant hymen visualized using labial separation. Hymenal tissue is pale and avascular with multiple overlapping folds of tissue.

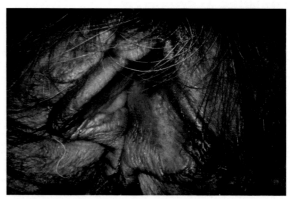

Figure 3-29
Labia majora and labia minora of postmenopausal woman. Note decreased genital elasticity and loss of adipose tissue associated with a decrease in endogenous estrogen production.

2006). The hymen becomes redundant, thick (Myhre, Myklestad, Adams, 2010), pale, elastic, and nontender as depicted in Figure 3-28. Due to the redundant nature of the hymenal tissue associated with puberty and childbearing years, alternative methods including sterile water irrigation or the use of a cotton swab or Foley catheter are frequently required to adequately assess the hymenal rim for findings.

As females progress toward menopause, endogenous estrogen levels begin to decline. In the absence of estrogen replacement therapy, the genitalia of postmenopausal females become atrophied and thin with a subsequent decrease of adipose tissue and elasticity as depicted in Figures 3-29, 3-30, and 3-31. The **columnar epithelium** responsible for cervical ectropion tissue

is no longer visible as it transitions into the cervical canal. As the vaginal pH changes from acidic to basic, vaginal discharge and lubrication decrease (Basaran, Kosif, Bayar, Civelek, 2008; Farage, Maibach, 2006; Kelley, 2007).

TANNER STAGES

Tanner staging is a means of standardizing the assessment of secondary sex characteristics in both males and females. Tanner staging assesses breast and pubic hair development in females and penile, scrotal, testicular and pubic hair development in males. Refer to Figure 3-32 for female Tanner stages and Figure 3-33 for male Tanner stages (Ceo, 2006; Farage, Maibach, 2006).

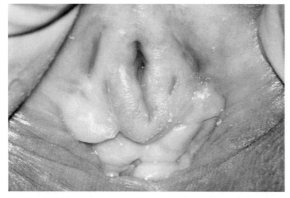

Figure 3-30
Pale, thin, atrophied labia minora, urethral os, and hymen associated with a decrease in endogenous estrogen; postmenopausal woman.

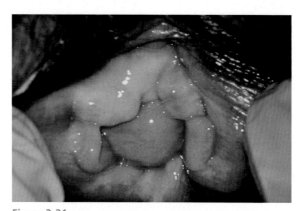

Figure 3-31
Postmenopausal woman; pale, atrophied hymen associated with a decrease in endogenous estrogen; cystocele visible.

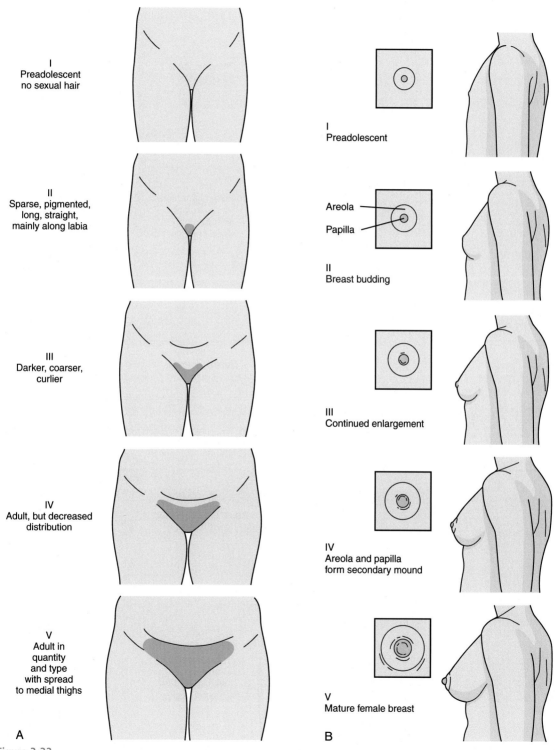

I
Preadolescent
no sexual hair

II
Sparse, pigmented,
long, straight,
mainly along labia

III
Darker, coarser,
curlier

IV
Adult, but decreased
distribution

V
Adult in
quantity
and type
with spread
to medial thighs

A

I
Preadolescent

Areola
Papilla

II
Breast budding

III
Continued enlargement

IV
Areola and papilla
form secondary mound

V
Mature female breast

B

Figure 3-32
Female Tanner Stages of growth and development. (From Zitelli, B. (2007). *Atlas of pediatric physical diagnosis.* (5th ed.). Philadelphia: Mosby.)

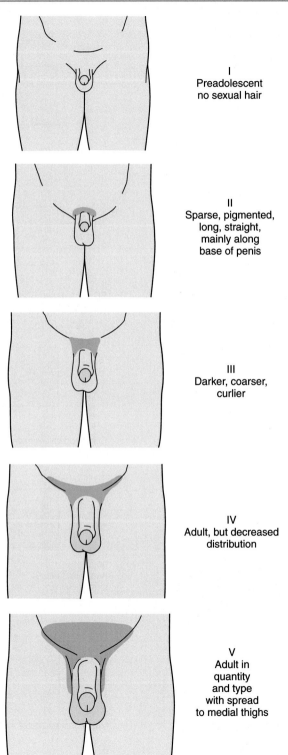

I
Preadolescent
no sexual hair

II
Sparse, pigmented,
long, straight,
mainly along
base of penis

III
Darker, coarser,
curlier

IV
Adult, but decreased
distribution

V
Adult in
quantity
and type
with spread
to medial thighs

Figure 3-33
Male Tanner Stages of growth and development. (From Zitelli, B. (2007). *Atlas of pediatric physical diagnosis*. (5th ed.). Philadelphia: Mosby.)

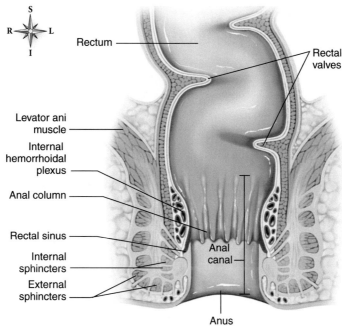

Figure 3-34
Anorectal anatomy. (From Patton K. T., & Thibodeau G. A. (2010). *Anatomy & physiology.* (7th ed.). St Louis, MO: Mosby.)

ANORECTAL ANATOMY

The **anorectal** canal is the distal most portion of the large intestine. Figure 3-34 identifies anal and rectal anatomical structures. The **rectum** has thin, pink to salmon colored mucosa (Figures 3-35 and 3-36), is approximately 12 to 18 cm in length and functions to collect and hold stool prior to defecation. The anal canal is approximately 2.5 to 5 cm long and includes the internal and external anal sphincters, which are responsible for regulating bowel continence and the passage of stool (Barleben, Mills, 2010). The **external anal sphincter** is composed of skeletal muscle and is under voluntary control in the absence of neuromuscular disorders, sedation or other forms of altered mental status. The **internal anal sphincter** is composed of involuntary smooth muscle (Ellis, 2010; Marieb, 2006). With pending defecation, the rectal reservoir becomes distended causing relaxation of the internal anal sphincter. Contraction of the external anal sphincter

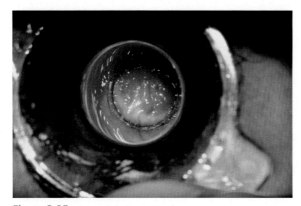

Figure 3-35
Normal rectum visualized using an anoscope.

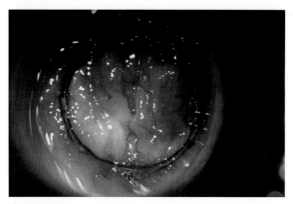

Figure 3-36
Normal rectum visualized using an anoscope.

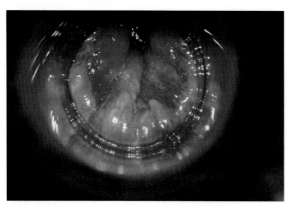

Figure 3-37
Dentate (also known as pectinate) line visualized with an anoscope.

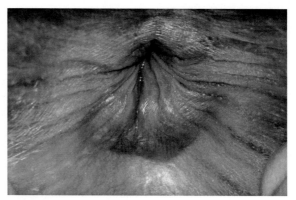

Figure 3-38
Venous pooling. Note the bluish-red discoloration and swelling associated with prolonged separation of the perianal tissue.

maintains continence until inhibiting stimulation from the nervous system allows relaxation and stool passage (Barleben, Mills, 2010; Bharucha, 2006).

The proximal anal canal is composed of columnar epithelium while the distal anal canal is composed of stratified epithelium (Bharucha, 2006). The intersection between these two types of tissues form the anal transitional zone also known as the dentate or **pectinate line.** The saw-toothed appearance of the **dentate line** (Figure 3-37) is created by alternating folds of mucosal tissue that form the anal columns and the alternating spaces, which are referred to as the anal crypts or sinuses (Barleben, Mills, 2010).

The anal canal terminates in the **anus** (Marieb, 2006). Prolonged separation of the perianal tissue during visual inspections frequently results in venous congestion or pooling. Figures 3-38 and 3-39 depict the typical bluish to red discoloration and perianal swelling associated with venous pooling. **Venous pooling** should not be misinterpreted as a traumatic finding. Allowing the patient to relax and change positions prior to re-examining the anus will result in resolution of this normal finding.

The anal verge is the transformation zone between the internal anal **squamous epithelium** and the keratinized epithelium that comprises the external anal folds. The perianal folds or rugae are created by the external anal sphincter and radiate outward from the anus as indicated by Figure 3-40. The anal rugae flatten when the external anal sphincter relaxes during defecation.

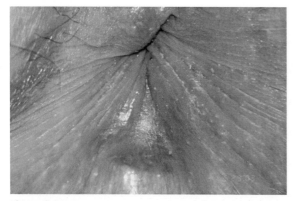

Figure 3-39
Venous pooling. Bluish-red discoloration and swelling should not be mistaken for perianal bruising and swelling associated with trauma.

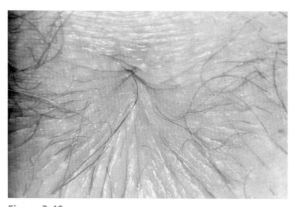

Figure 3-40
Perianal folds radiate outward from the anus and are created by contraction of the external anal sphincter.

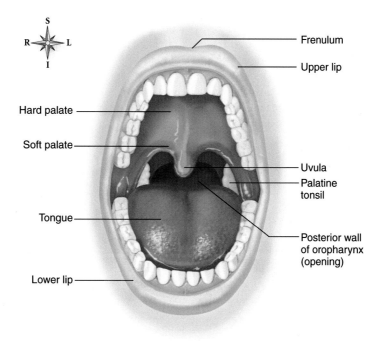

Figure 3-41
Oral cavity anatomy. (From Patton K. T., & Thibodeau G. A. (2010). *Anatomy & physiology.* (7th ed.). St Louis, MO: Mosby.)

ORAL ANATOMY

The **oral cavity** comprises the lips, cheeks or buccal mucosa, hard and soft palates, the tongue, several frenula, the uvula, oropharynx, dentition, **gingiva** or gums, and tonsils as indicated by Figures 3-41 and 3-42. The lips are composed of keratinized tissue externally, non-keratinized tissue internally and provide protection to the oral cavity. The lips are attached internally to the gingiva by two frenula, one upper and one lower. The cheeks or **buccal mucosa** are composed of non-keratinized mucosal tissue and are the site for obtaining source DNA specimens or buccal swabs. The hard and soft palates form the roof of the mouth. The **hard palate** is anterior to the **soft palate.** The tongue is composed of muscular tissue with several bony attachment points and is attached to the floor of the oral cavity by the lingual **frenulum.** The tongue is covered by papillae, which contain taste receptors. The **uvula** extends downward from the posterior aspect of the soft palate. There are two sets of tonsils located in the oral cavity; the palatine tonsils, which are located

in the posterior aspect of the oral cavity and the lingual tonsils, which are located at the base of the tongue. The **tonsils** are composed of lymphatic tissue and function by protecting the body from infectious processes. The **oropharynx** is the posterior aspect of the oral cavity. The **dentition** is composed of two sets of teeth, the deciduous and the permanent teeth.

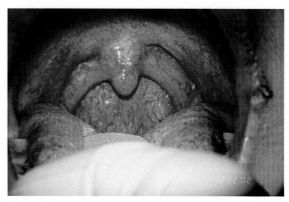

Figure 3-42
Oropharynx.

By the age of two, the deciduous or baby teeth have erupted until the age of six to twelve when they begin to loosen and fall out. By the end of adolescence, the permanent teeth have fully erupted with the exception of the wisdom teeth, which may or may not erupt by the age of 25. Each tooth is composed of a root, a crown, and pulp. The exposed portion of the tooth, the crown, is composed of dentin internally and enamel externally. The root of each tooth extends under the gingiva where it is anchored in the jaw. The internal cavity of each tooth contains pulp, which is composed of connective tissue, blood vessels and nerves (Marieb, 2006).

ANATOMICAL VARIANTS

There are numerous normal anatomical variants of the oral anatomy and the female and male anogenital structures. Forensic examiners should seek additional resources and education to become proficient in identifying these normal anatomical variants to prevent misinterpreting oral and anogenital findings seen during sexual assault examinations.

Key Terms

Accessory glands
Adipose tissue
Annular
Anorectal
Anterior commissure
Anus
Atrophic
Bartholin gland
Buccal mucosa
Bulbourethral gland
Cervix
Clitoris
Columnar epithelium
Corpora cavernosa
Corpus spongiosum
Cowper gland
Crescentic hymen
Cribiform hymen
Cystocele
Dentate line
Dentition
Ejaculation
Epididymis
Estrogen

External anal sphincter
External genitalia
Fallopian tubes
Fimbriated hymen
Foreskin
Fossa navicularis
Frenulum
Gingiva
Glans
Hard palate
Hymen
Imperforate hymen
Internal anal sphincter
Labia majora
Labia minora
Longitudinal ridge
Mons pubis
Oral cavity
Oropharynx
Ovaries
Pectinate line
Penile shaft
Penis
Perineum
Posterior fourchette
Postmenopause
Prepuce
Prostate gland
Puberty
Rectocele
Rectum
Scrotum
Sebaceous glands
Seminiferous tubules
Septate
Skene gland
Soft palate
Spermatozoa
Squamous epithelium
Sudoriferous glands
Symphysis pubis
Tanner staging
Testes
Testosterone
Tonsils
Transverse folds
Urethra
Uterus

Uvula
Vagina
Vaginal columns
Vaginal introitus
Vaginal rugae
Vas deferens
Venous pooling
Vestibule
Vulva

References

Barleben, A., & Mills, S. (2010). Anorectal anatomy and physiology. *Surgical Clinics North America, 90,* 1–15.

Basaran, M., Kosif, R., Bayar, U., & Civelek, B. (2008). Characteristics of external genitalia in pre- and postmenopausal women. *Climacteric, 11,* 416–421.

Berek, J. S., & Novak, E. (2007). *Berek & Novak's Gynecology.* (14th ed.). Philadelphia: Lippincott, Williams & Wilkins.

Berenson, A. B. (1995). A longitudinal study of hymenal morphology in the first 3 years of life. *Pediatrics, 95* (4), 490–496.

Berenson, A. B. (1998). Normal anogenital anatomy. *Child Abuse and Neglect, 22* (6), 589–596.

Bharucha, A. E. (2006). Pelvic floor: Anatomy and function. *Neurogastroenterology and Motility, 18,* 507–519.

Bikoo, M. (2007). Female genital mutilation: Classification and management. *Nursing Standard, 22* (7), 43–49.

Ceo, P. D. (2006). Assessment of the male reproductive system. *Urologic Nursing, 26* (4), 290–296.

Ellis, H. (2010). The applied anatomy of rectal examination. *British Journal of Hospital Medicine, 71* (9), M132–M133.

Farage, M., & Maibach, H. (2006). Lifetime changes in the vulva and vagina. *Archives of Gynecology & Obstetrics, 273,* 195–202.

Heger, A. H., Ticson, L., Guerra, L., et al. (2002). Appearance of the genitalia in girls selected for nonabuse: Review of hymenal morphology and nonspecific findings. *Journal of Pediatric and Adolescent Gynecology, 15,* 27–35.

Hobday, A. J., Haury, L., & Dayton, P. K. (1997). Function of the human hymen. *Medical Hypotheses, 49,* 171–173.

Kelley, C. (2007). Estrogen and its effect on vaginal atrophy in post-menopausal women. *Urology Nursing, 27* (1), 40–45.

Kochhar, R., Taylor, B., & Sangar, V. (2010). Imaging in primary penile cancer: Current status and future directions. *European Radiology, 20,* 36–47.

Lawton, S., & Littlewood, S. (2006). Vulval skin disease: Clinical features, assessment and management. *Nursing Standard, 20* (42), 57–63.

Marieb, E. N. (2006). *Essentials of Human Anatomy & Physiology.* (8th ed.). San Francisco: Pearson Education, Inc.

Matiluko, A. F. (2009). Cervical ectropion. Part 1: Appraisal of a common clinical finding. *Trends in Urology, Gynaecology & Sexual Health, 14* (3), 10–12.

McCann, J., Wells, R., Simon, M. D., & Voris, J. (1990). Genital findings in prepubertal girls selected for nonabuse: A descriptive study. *Pediatrics, 86* (3), 428–439.

Myhre, A. K., Myklestad, K., & Adams, J. A. (2010). Changes in genital anatomy and microbiology in girls between age 6 and age 12 years: A longitudinal study. *North American Society for Pediatric and Adolescent Gynecology, 23,* 77–85.

Nucci, M. R., & Oliva, E. (2009). *Gynecologic Pathology.* Philadelphia: Elsevier Churchill Livingstone.

Ostrzenski, A. (2002). Gynecology: *Integrating conventional, complementary, and natural alternative therapy.* Philadelphia: Lippincott, Williams & Wilkins.

Perry-Philo, D., & Bradford, J. L. (2007). *Understanding Medical Surgical Nursing,* (3rd ed.). Philadelphia: F.A. Davis Company.

Puppo, V. (2011). Embryology and anatomy of the vulva: The female orgasm and women's sexual health. *European Journal of Obstetrics & Gynecology and Reproductive Biology, 154,* 3–8.

Yang, C. C., Cold, C. J., Yilmaz, U., & Maravilla, K. R. (2005). Sexually responsive vascular tissue of the vulva. *BJU International, 97,* 766–772.

CHAPTER 4

ANOGENITAL DERMATOLOGY

Tara Henry

Medical-forensic evaluation of the anogenitalia requires knowledge and recognition of normal anatomic structures and epithelia. This chapter will provide an overview of some commonly misinterpreted normal findings and discuss some abnormal findings, which could be confused with trauma or associated with trauma due to underlying pathology. Anogenital trauma will be discussed in other chapters of this text.

SKIN ANATOMY

Skin has three layers (Figure 4-1). The top outermost layer is the **epidermis**, also called the cutaneous layer. It is composed of stratified squamous epithelial cells and does not contain blood vessels or nerve endings. Although the epidermis is only a

few cell layers thick, 0.05 to 1.5 mm (Habif, 2009), it has many functions.

> The epidermis provides protection from harmful substances such as heat, chemicals, microbes, and ultraviolet radiation. It preserves the internal environment of the body by preventing the loss of water, electrolytes, and macromolecules such as protein (Weller, Hunter, Savin, Dahl, 2008).

These functions are performed by four cell types in the epidermis. **Keratinocytes,** which make up approximately 85% of the epidermis, produce keratin that protects the skin. **Melanocytes** synthesize melanin and are responsible for skin pigmentation and protection

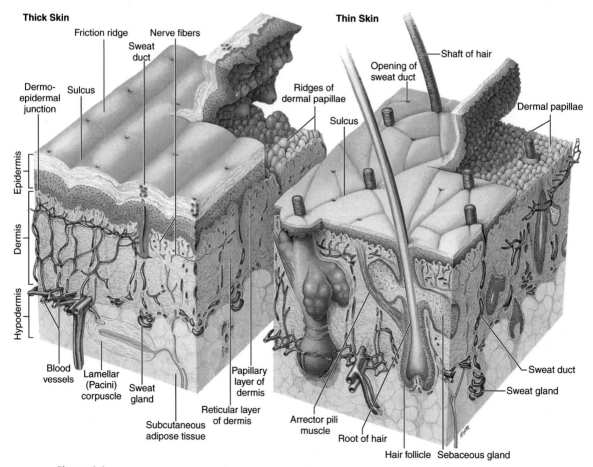

Figure 4-1
Structure of the skin. (From Patton K. T., & Thibodeau G. A. (2010). *Anatomy & physiology.* (7th ed.). St Louis, MO: Mosby.)

from ultraviolet radiation. **Langerhans cells** are responsible for the immune reaction of the skin and Merkel's cells act as transducers for fine touch (Weller, Hunter, Savin, Dahl, 2008).

The mid layer is the **dermis**. It lies beneath the epidermis, varies from 1 to 4 mm thick and is composed of collagen-rich connective tissue, elastic tissue, and reticular fibers. The dermis has an abundant blood and nerve supply, hair follicles, and sweat and oil glands.

> The dermis acts as a shock absorber, providing the skin with strength, extensibility, and elasticity (Patton, Thibodeau, 2010). It helps regulate body temperature and is the key layer for achieving proper wound repair (Trott, 2005).

The bottom layer is the subcutaneous layer, also known as the superficial fascia. It is composed of loose connective tissue and adipose tissue (fat) and is the layer that helps determine the shape of the body.

> The subcutaneous layer stores energy and insulates the body.

TERMINOLOGY OF SKIN LESIONS
PRIMARY LESIONS

> A **primary skin lesion** develops on unaltered skin as a direct result of a disease process. For primary lesions, it is the size of the lesion that determines the term the healthcare provider uses to describe the lesion.

A flat area of discoloration measuring less than 1 cm is a **macule** (e.g., freckle, hypopigmentation); larger than 1 cm is a **patch** (e.g., Mongolian spot, vitiligo). A superficial elevated solid lesion less than 1 cm is a **papule** (e.g., mole, wart); larger than 1 cm is a **plaque** (e.g., psoriasis, eczema). A **nodule** is also an elevated solid lesion, larger than 1 cm, however it extends deeper into the dermis than a papule (e.g., fibroma, xanthoma). An elevated collection of free fluid less than 1 cm is a **vesicle** (e.g., herpes simplex, herpes zoster); larger than

1 cm is a **bulla** (e.g., burn, friction blister). An elevated collection of turbid fluid (leukocytes and free fluid) less than 1 cm is a **pustule** (e.g., acne, impetigo); larger than 1 cm is an **abscess** (e.g., furuncle, carbuncle). A superficial, transitory, edematous plaque caused from infiltration of the dermis with fluid is a **wheal** (e.g., bee sting, allergic reaction). Wheals can be any size and are often very pruritic (Weller, et al., 2008; Patton, 2008).

SECONDARY LESIONS

> **Secondary lesions** evolve from primary lesions due to the evolution of the lesion, passage of time, scratching, or infection.

Scales are silvery or white flakes of skin that may be dry or greasy and are caused by the shedding of dead excess keratinocytes. A **crust** is a collection of dried serum left after vesicles or pustules rupture and dry, or after lacerations and abrasions dry. **Erosions** are a superficial loss of epidermis that are moist but without bleeding, and do not scar when they heal; whereas **ulcers** are a deeper loss of epidermis and dermis, may bleed, and do leave a scar when they heal. **Excoriations** refer to superficial linear abrasions usually self-inflicted as a result of intense itching or chaffing. Fissures are linear cracks or splits that extend into the dermis. Skin that is chronically moist may have superficial linear cracks or splits, which are referred to as macerations. **Lichenification** is an area of thickened, leathery skin with exaggeration of normal skin markings. **Scars** are permanent fibrotic changes that occur as the normal tissue is replaced with collagen-rich connective tissue when the skin lesion or injury heals. (Weller, Hunter, Savin, Dahl, 2008; Habif, 2009).

HISTORY AND PHYSICAL EXAMINATION

> It is important for forensic examiners to have knowledge about normal anogenital variants and common anogenital dermatological conditions to prevent misdiagnoses of trauma, identify differential diagnoses of anogenital findings, and provide appropriate treatment or referrals for further care after the medical-forensic examination.

A careful history and physical examination are needed for accurate diagnosis and treatment of anogenital dermatological conditions. The medical history should include onset and duration of anogenital symptoms, any associated non-genital symptoms, pertinent sexual history, prior treatment for anogenital conditions, other medical problems, and medications including over-the-counter drugs. The physical examination of the anogenitalia includes identification of any primary lesions and/or any secondary changes that have occurred. Additional assessment of the lesions should consist of the size, color, sharpness and characteristics of the edge, surface contour, shape, texture, distribution, configuration, smell, and temperature (Weller, Hunter, Savin, Dahl, 2008; Jarvis, 2008). See Table 4-1 for examples of common descriptors.

NORMAL VARIANTS

There are many normal variants of the anogenital anatomy. Forensic examiners should observe and recognize normal variant findings for each patient. Genital epithelium is known to have more pigment than skin elsewhere on the body. As a result, the color of external genital skin may present as darker than expected in some patients.

Mild redness of the vulva and vaginal walls is normal and varies from patient to patient (Figure 4-2). Care should be taken not to misinterpret this redness as trauma or inflammation.

Physiologic hyperpigmentation is common, particularly with darker complexions. It is generally located on the labia minora and perineum (Figures 4-3). **Postinflammatory hyperpigmentation** may occur after trauma or chronic inflammatory conditions. This type of hyperpigmentation is seen as irregular light to dark brown macules or patches at the location of the trauma or inflammatory condition (Figure 4-4). The most common hyperpigmentation of the vulvar skin is lentigo simplex. **Lentigo simplex** are benign macules caused by excess melanin production. They are located on the labia majora or labia minora, but they do not

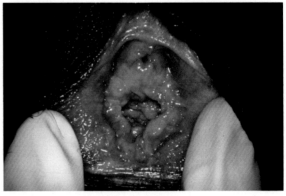

Figure 4-2
Normal generalized redness of vestibule.

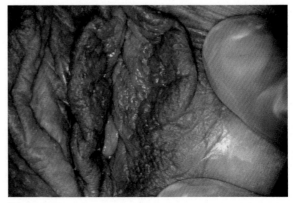

Figure 4-3
Physiologic hyperpigmentation of labia minora.

TABLE 4-1	Common Dermatologic Descriptors	
Shapes	**Configuration**	**Contours**
Annular	Confluent	Acuminata
Arcuate	Dermatomal	Dome-shaped
Circinate	Discrete	Flat-topped
Discoid	Grouped	Pedunculated
Gyrate	Linear	Umbilicated
Nummular	Segmented	Verrucous
Polycyclic	Serpiginous	
Reticulate		
Targetoid		

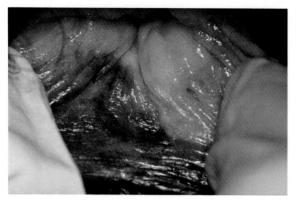

Figure 4-4
Postinflammatory hyperpigmentation of the fossa navicularis.

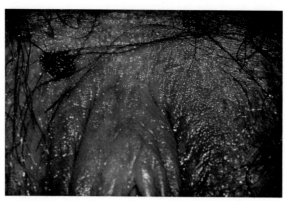

Figure 4-5
Lentigo simplex on labia majora.

involve the mucous membrane area. They are brown, with irregular borders, and are uniformly pigmented (Figure 4-5). Another form of hyperpigmentation caused by an excess production of melanin is genital **melanosis**. Unlike lentigo simplex, genital melanosis can involve the mucous membrane of the vulva. They are irregular, poorly demarcated, brown to black macules or patches that are more than 4 mm in dimension (Figure 4-6) (Edwards, 2010; Wilkinson, Stone, 2008).

Nevi, also known as melanocytic nevi, are benign skin tumors that are symmetrical macules or papules, smaller than 10 mm in diameter, with well-defined borders, and uniformly pigmented brown in color (Figures 4-7 to 4-9) (Wilkinson, Stone, 2008). Atypical nevi are generally greater than 6 mm, asymmetrical, with irregular borders, and have a variety of colors. Melanomas are malignant nevi that have irregular

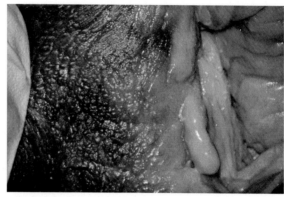

Figure 4-6
Genital melanosis on right labium minus.

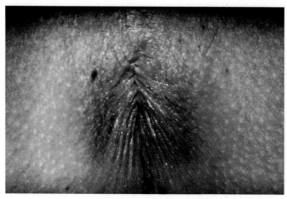

Figure 4-7
Melanocytic nevi on perianal area and buttocks.

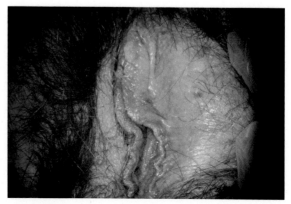

Figure 4-8
Melanocytic nevi on left labium majus and left labium minus.

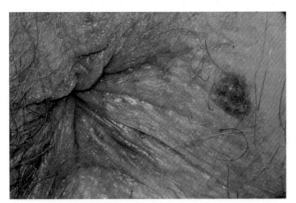

Figure 4-9
Melanocytic nevi on perianal area at the 3 o'clock position.

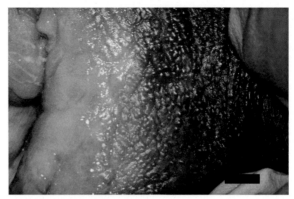

Figure 4-10
Vestibular papilla on right labium minus.

borders and color variegation. They are often dark brown or black, but can be red, blue, grey, white, or amelanotic (Edwards, 2010).

> Any suspected atypical nevi or melanoma identified during a medical-forensic sexual assault examination requires a referral for further evaluation.

Vestibular papillae are soft, filliform, tubular structures found on the inner labia minora and occasionally on the labia minora edges. They are symmetric in distribution, can occur in patches or be confluent, and have a cobblestone appearance (Figures 4-10 and 4-11). Care should be taken not to mistake vestibular papillae for genital warts. Genital warts tend to have a broader, fused base and have a denser consistency,

whereas vestibular papillae are delicate structures with discreet bases.

Pearly penile papules are small, skin color, white to pink papules that occur in rows around the edge of the corona of the glans penis. The papules vary in size from less than 1 mm to 3 mm. They are more prominent in uncircumcised males. These are a normal anatomic variant and should not be mistaken for genital warts.

Fordyce's spots are enlarged sebaceous glands, visible through the thin epithelium of the labia minora, particularly the medial aspect. Fordyce's spots are white to yellow in color and can be made more apparent by gently stretching the labia minora (Figures 4-12 and 4-13) (Edwards, 2010). These can also be mistaken for genital warts; therefore, recognition of this normal variant is important. Fordyce's spots may also

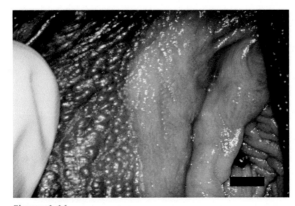

Figure 4-11
Vestibular papilla on left labium minus.

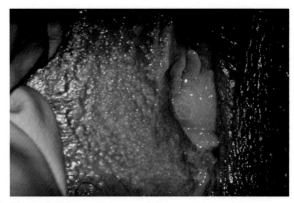

Figure 4-12
Fordyce's spots on right labium minus.

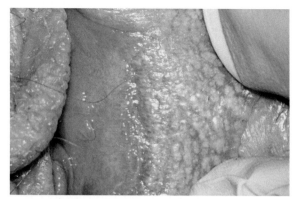

Figure 4-13
Fordyce's spots on left labium minus.

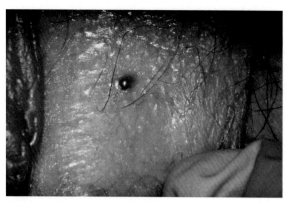

Figure 4-14
Angiokeratoma on left labium minus.

be seen in males, becoming visible when the penile skin is thinned by stretching or during erection.

Angiokeratomas are benign vascular papules that occur most often on the labia majora or scrotum. They are 2 to 5 mm in diameter, range in color from black to dark red to purple, are nontender, and usually multiple in number (Figures 4-14 and 4-15) (Wilkinson, Stone, 2008).

> Care should be taken not to mistake angiokeratomas for bruising, blood filled vesicles, or hematomas.

Cherry angiomas are another benign vascular lesion seen on the genitalia. These are bright or deep red, usually flat pinpoint lesions, but can be up to 4 mm in diameter (Figure 4-16) (Edwards, 2010). They are nontender and do not blanch.

> **Cherry angiomas** can be mistaken for petechiae, especially by lesser experienced forensic examiners.

COMMON ANOGENITAL CONDITIONS

Folliculitis is an inflammation of the hair follicle. It can be caused by organisms such as *Staphylococcus aureus* or result from noninfectious causes like shaving, waxing, or plucking of hairs. Folliculitis lesions may be singular or multiple and present as red papules or pustules. These lesions may or may not be tender (Figure 4-17).

Hidradenitis suppurativa is caused by occlusion of the hair follicle that results in the obstruction and inflammation of the apocrine glands. It is considered

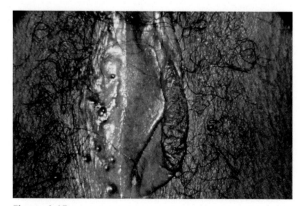

Figure 4-15
Multiple angiokeratomas on labia majora.

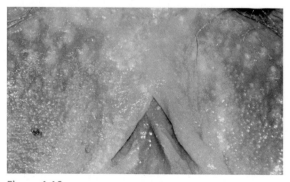

Figure 4-16
Cherry angioma on right labia major.

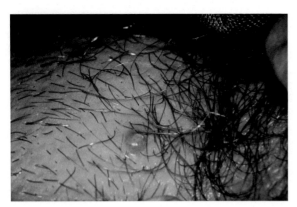

Figure 4-17
Folliculitis on right side of mons pubis.

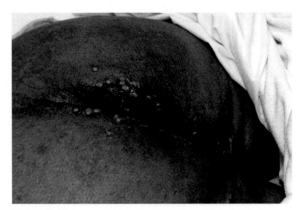

Figure 4-18
Hidradenitis suppurativa on buttocks.

to be the equivalent of cystic acne (Edwards, 2010). Hidradenitis suppurativa presents as painful, red nodules and comedomes that progress to abscesses and sinus tracts (Figure 4-18). This is a chronic disease; therefore, the examiner should expect to see evidence of recurrent draining nodules, sinus tracts, and scars.

Mucous cysts are benign, asymptomatic cysts that result from an obstruction of the vestibular glands. They occur on the medial aspect of the labia minora, can be up to 3 cm in diameter from the build-up of debris, and range from skin color to yellowish or blue (Figures 4-19 and 4-20) (Edwards, 2010). Depending on the location, mucous cysts can be confused with Skene gland cysts or Bartholin gland cysts. When bluish in color, lesser experienced examiners may mistake them for hematomas.

Bartholin gland cysts result from an occlusion of the Bartholin gland ducts. They are located at the 5 o'clock and the 7 o'clock positions on the labia minora, are skin color, have diffuse swelling, and are usually asymptomatic. When traumatized or infected, they become red and painful abscesses (Figures 4-21 and 4-22). Bartholin gland cysts and abscesses are most often unilateral; however, they can be bilateral.

Skene duct cysts result from an obstruction of the Skene gland ducts. They are visible at the urethral meatus, less than 1 cm in diameter, nontender, and usually asymptomatic unless infected. Occasionally the patient may report changes in urinary stream, dysuria or dyspareunia (Wilkinson, Stone, 2008).

Epidermal inclusion cysts are benign cysts thought to be a result of implantation of the epidermis

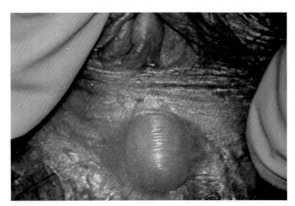

Figure 4-19
Mucous cyst below clitoris on labia minora.

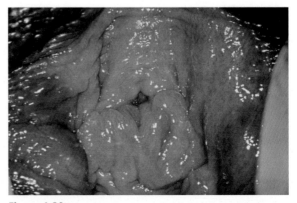

Figure 4-20
Mucous cysts on labia minora at the 3 o'clock and the 9 o'clock positions. Should not be confused with Bartholin gland cysts, which would be located at the 5 o'clock and the 7 o'clock positions.

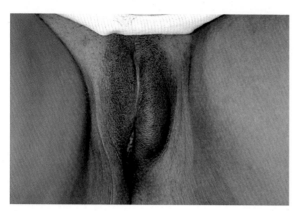

Figure 4-21
Infected left Bartholin gland.

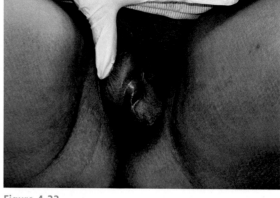

Figure 4-22
Right labial abscess.

within the dermis, probably secondary to trauma (Wilkinson, Stone, 2008). They can also be formed by an obstructed or malformed hair follicle (Edwards, 2010). Typically they are asymptomatic, smooth, mobile, skin color to slightly yellow nodules (Figure 4-23). Some epidermal cysts have keratin plugs, which present as a black-colored opening that produces a cheese-like, foul smelling, yellowish discharge when pressed.

> The cervix is lined with many glands that release mucous. Occlusion of these glands results in mucous filled **nabothian cysts** on the surface of the cervix.

They present as smooth, rounded bumps, which may be singular or multiple (Figures 4-24 and 4-25). The cysts are benign, nontender, and asymptomatic.

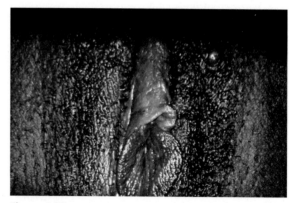

Figure 4-23
Small epidermal inclusion cyst on left labium majus.

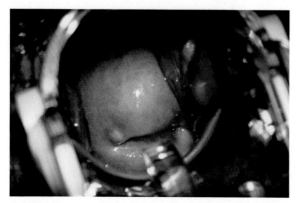

Figure 4-24
Nabothian cyst on cervix at the 9 o'clock position.

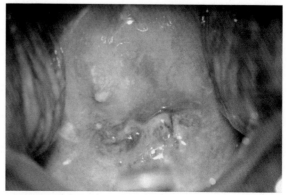

Figure 4-25
Multiple nabothian cysts on cervix.

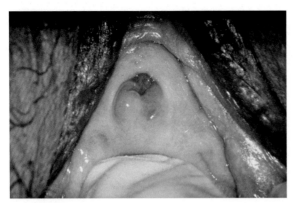

Figure 4-26
Urethral caruncle.

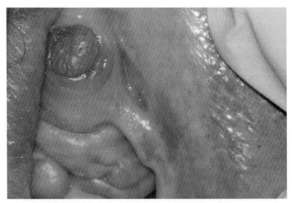

Figure 4-27
Urethral prolapse.

Urethral caruncles are small benign outgrowths of the distal urethral mucosa (Figure 4-26). They are generally seen in postmenopausal women. Symptoms can range from asymptomatic to painful, bleeding, or dysuria. **Urethral prolapses** resemble caruncles in appearance. Prolapses tend to be less symptomatic and usually are circumferential around the meatus when they are complete (Figure 4-27).

Lichen sclerosis is a chronic inflammatory condition that results in epithelial thinning, dermal changes, and inflammation (Wilkinson, Stone, 2008). The classic presentation consists of white patches in an hourglass or figure-eight pattern on the labia majora, labia minora, perineum, and perianal area and on any part of the penis, most often on the glans and prepuce (Edwards, 2010). The skin is atrophic and fragile, often having areas of ecchymosis or hyperpigmentation that can be mistaken for trauma by examiners unfamiliar with this condition. Other symptoms associated with lichen sclerosis are pruritis, burning, and painful intercourse.

COMMON INFECTIOUS ANOGENITAL CONDITIONS

Bacterial vaginosis is caused by an overgrowth of anaerobic bacteria, which deplete the hydrogen peroxide producing *Lactobacillus* in the vagina. It is associated with having multiple male or female partners, a new sex partner, douching, lack of condom use, and lack of vaginal lactobacilli. Although bacterial vaginosis is associated with sexual activity, women who have never had sex can also be affected (Centers for Disease Control and Prevention (CDC), 2010). Symptoms include homogenous, milky discharge that coats vaginal walls and/or labia minora and a "fishy" odor (Figures 4-28 and 4-29).

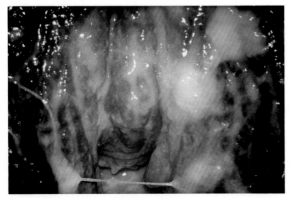

Figure 4-28
White homogenous discharge from bacterial vaginosis.

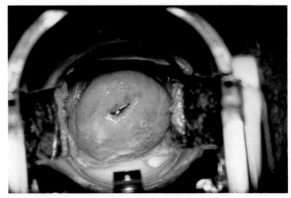

Figure 4-29
Thin white homogenous discharge in vaginal vault from bacterial vaginosis.

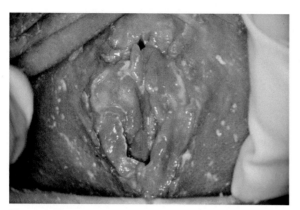

Figure 4-30
White, clumped vaginal discharge from candidiasis.

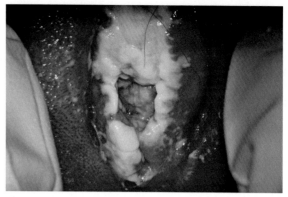

Figure 4-31
White adherent vaginal discharge from candidiasis. Note bright red vestibule irritation.

Diagnosis requires three of the following four criteria to be met: thin, white, homogenous malodorous, adherent vaginal discharge; pH over 4.5; positive whiff test; and presence of clue cells by wet-mount microscopy.

Diagnosis is made by wet-mount microscopy or Gram stain of the vaginal discharge that demonstrates yeasts, hyphae, or pseudohyphae; or by culture (Hainer, Gibson, 2011).

Candidiasis is caused by an overgrowth of *Candida,* usually *Candida albicans,* in the vagina as a result of a homeostatic imbalance of the normal vaginal flora. It is associated with antibiotic use, obesity, diabetes, and pregnancy. Symptoms include dysuria and pruritis. When present, vaginal discharge is thick, white, clumped, and adherent (Figures 4-30 to 4-32). Other signs may include labial and vaginal redness, swelling, and excoriations.

Trichomoniasis is a sexually transmitted infection caused by the parasite *Trichomonas vaginalis.* Symptoms include yellow to green vaginal discharge that can be bubbly and foul smelling (Figure 4-33). Pruritis, dysuria, and dyspareunia can occur, but often men and women are asymptomatic. Other signs include redness and swelling of the vulva or petechial lesions on the cervix, otherwise known as "strawberry cervix" (Figure 4-34).

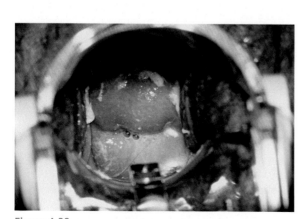

Figure 4-32
Thick, white, clumped vaginal discharge from candidiasis.

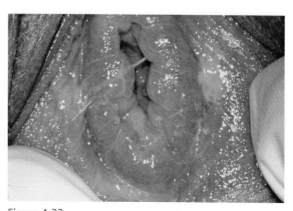

Figure 4-33
Yellow-tinged vaginal discharge from trichomoniasis.

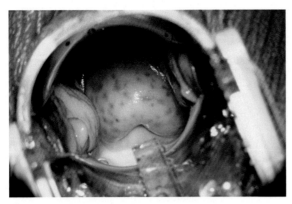

Figure 4-34
"Strawberry cervix" from trichomoniasis.

Diagnosis is made by wet-mount microscopy, OSOM® Trichomonas Rapid Test, Affirm VP III, or culture (CDC, 2010; Hainer, Gibson, 2011).

Chlamydia trachomatis is the most common bacterial sexually transmitted infection worldwide (WHO, 2011).

Chlamydial genital infections are frequently asymptomatic. When symptoms are present, men have urethral discharge and dysuria; women have vaginal discharge, dysuria, spotting between menses or during sex, or lower abdominal pain. The cervix may show mucopurulent discharge, cervical ectopy; friability (Figures 4-35 and 4-36), or cervical motion tenderness.

Left untreated, Chlamydial infections in women can progress to pelvic inflammatory disease, infertility or ectopic pregnancies.

Diagnosis is made by urine testing, culture, nucleic acid amplification tests (NAAT), or nucleic acid hybridization tests.

Neisseria gonorrhoeae is the second most commonly reported bacterial sexually transmitted infection in the United States (CDC, 2010). Men are symptomatic with urethral discharge and dysuria. Women are often asymptomatic until complications arise such as pelvic inflammatory disease.

When symptoms are present, women can have purulent endocervical discharge, ectopy, and friability (Figure 4-37). Symptoms of rectal infection include purulent discharge and rectal mucosa redness. Pharyngeal infections are usually asymptomatic; however, if present, include pharyngeal redness, purulent exudate, and cervical lymphadenopathy.

Diagnosis is made by urine testing, culture, NAAT, or nucleic acid hybridization tests.

Molluscum contagiosum *virus* is related to the pox virus. It is predominantly seen on the genitalia, abdomen, thighs, or buttocks. Molluscum lesions are small, pink- to skin-color, waxy, nontender papules with a central umbilication (Figures 4-38 and 4-39). These can be mistaken for genital warts, herpes, and folliculitis.

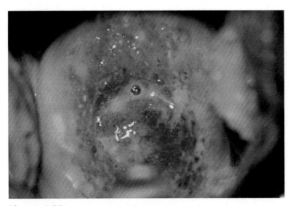

Figure 4-35
Thin, yellow discharge from Chlamydia. Note red, friable cervical ectopy.

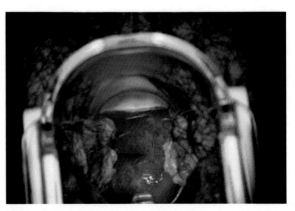

Figure 4-36
Scant amount of thin yellow discharge from Chlamydia. Note normal appearing cervix.

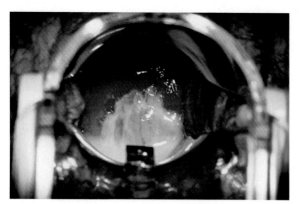

Figure 4-37
Thick purulent cervical discharge from Gonorrhea.

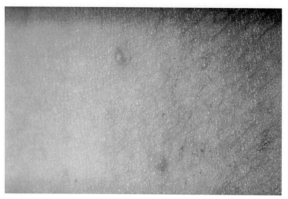

Figure 4-38
Molluscum on right labium majus. Note central umbilicus.

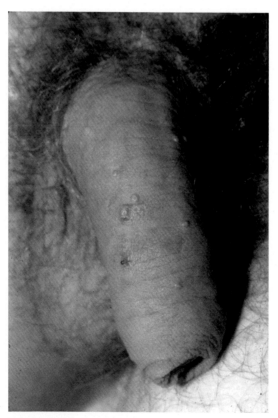

Figure 4-39
Molluscum on penis. Note central umbilicus.

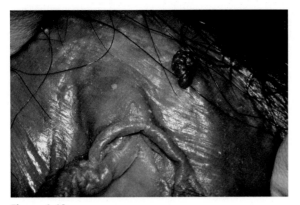

Figure 4-40
Genital wart on the left labium majus.

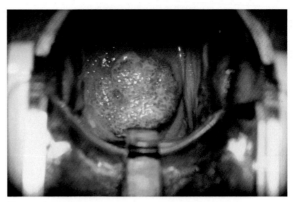

Figure 4-41
Genital warts on the cervix.

Genital warts are caused by the *human papilloma virus.* They are usually asymptomatic, but can produce itching and pain when irritated (CDC, 2010). Genital warts have a variety of morphology.

They can be single or multiple; round, pointed, or thin and slender; skin-color, pink, or white papules (Figures 4-40 to 4-44). When clustered together they have a cauliflower-like, verrucous, or plaque appearance (Edwards, 2010).

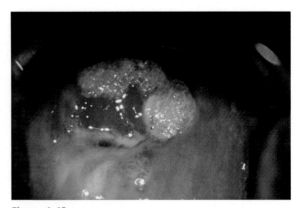

Figure 4-42
Genital warts on the cervix.

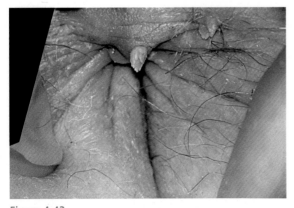

Figure 4-43
Genital warts on the anus.

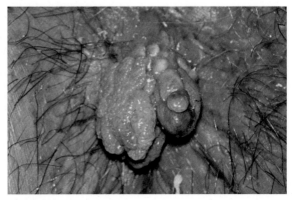

Figure 4-44
Genital warts on the anus.

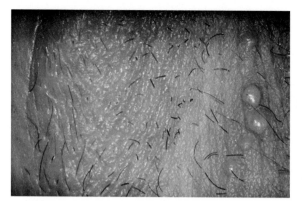

Figure 4-45
Herpes simplex vesicles on left labium majus.

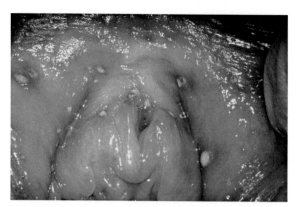

Figure 4-46
Ruptured herpes simplex vesicles, creating ulcers with surrounding redness in vestibule.

Genital herpes is caused by the *herpes simplex virus* (HSV). There are two types, HSV-1 and HSV-2. Both are chronic, lifelong viral infections (CDC, 2010).

The "classic" presentation of herpes is pruritis and burning sensation, followed by eruption of vesicles on the genitalia (Figure 4-45). The vesicles then rupture, resulting in ulcers (Figures 4-46 and 4-47).

Associated systemic symptoms of fever, headache, malaise, lymphadenopathy, dysuria, and urinary retention may occur, particularly with the initial outbreak (Edwards, 2010). Subsequent outbreaks of herpes are less painful and do not have systemic symptoms as often. Initial episodes of genital herpes infection do not always have the "classic" presentation; instead, the symptoms may be subclinical and the person may not be aware of the infection (Handsfield, 2001). Clinical diagnosis should be confirmed by virology or type-specific serologic testing (CDC, 2010).

Syphilis is caused by the bacterial spirochete *Treponema pallidum*. It is characterized by distinct primary, secondary, and tertiary stages that occur over several years or decades, interspersed by periods of latent infection (Handsfield, 2001). For the purpose of this chapter, only the primary stage of syphilis will be discussed.

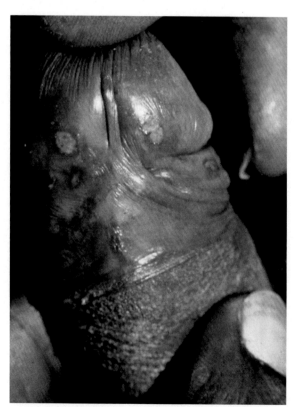

Figure 4-47
Ruptured herpes simplex vesicles on penis, creating ulcers with surrounding redness.

The primary stage of syphilis presents as a small, red papule that enlarges and ulcerates (Edwards, 2010) creating a painless, sharply demarcated, indurated chancre on the anogenitalia (Figures 4-48 and 4-49) (Wilkinson, Stone, 2008). The chancre is red, smooth, and without purulent exudate (Handsfield, 2001; Edwards, 2010).

Diagnosis of the chancre in the primary stages is made with darkfield microscopy. Serology is used to diagnose if the microscopy is negative, or after the primary stage has resolved (CDC, 2010).

PRACTICE IMPLICATIONS

Skin is the largest organ of the body with thousands of conditions that can affect it. Many non-genital skin conditions such as scabies, eczema, psoriasis, allergic drug reactions, among others can affect the anogenitalia.

Forensic examiners who perform medical-forensic sexual assault examinations should have a basic understanding of skin function, dermatology vocabulary, common skin conditions, and differential diagnoses for those conditions.

Trauma is just one of many conditions that impact the anogenital skin. It is important for forensic examiners to have the knowledge and skills to identify the anogenital findings that result from blunt and sharp force trauma. It is equally important for forensic examiners to consider alternate causes of the anogenital findings identified during the medical-forensic examination before diagnosing those findings as trauma. Many anogenital skin conditions make the tissue more susceptible to trauma. Forensic examiners must take this into consideration when determining factors that may influence the presence or absence of anogenital trauma from a reported sexual assault.

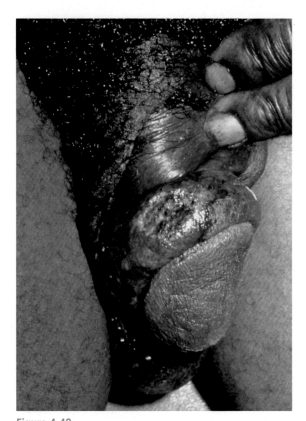

Figure 4-48
Syphilis chancre on the penis.

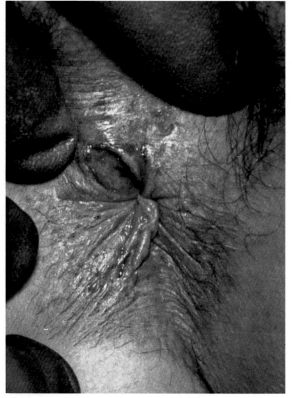

Figure 4-49
Syphilis chancre on the anus.

The ability to differentiate anogenital trauma from other chronic or acute anogenital skin conditions also allows the forensic examiner to initiate the appropriate treatment and/or referral to ensure the sexual assault patient's healthcare needs are addressed.

This chapter is meant to provide a basic introduction to anogenital dermatology. There are numerous textbooks, journals, online resources, and education opportunities via the dermatology, gynecology, infectious disease, and public health specialties that forensic examiners can utilize to improve their knowledge about various anogenital dermatologic conditions. In addition, forensic examiner educators should incorporate the more common dermatologic conditions into their basic and advanced sexual assault trainings and education.

Key Terms

Abscess
Angiokeratoma
Bacterial vaginosis
Bartholin gland cyst
Bulla
Candidiasis
Cherry angioma
Chlamydia trachomatis
Crust
Dermis
Epidermal inclusion cyst
Epidermis
Erosions
Excoriation
Folliculitis
Fordyce's spots
Genital herpes
Genital warts
Hidradenitis suppurativa
Keratinocytes
Langerhans cells
Lentigo simplex
Lichen sclerosis
Lichenification
Macule
Melanocyte

Melanosis
Molluscum contagiosum
Mucous cyst
Nabothian cyst
Neisseria gonorrhoeae
Nevi
Nodule
Papule
Patch
Pearly penile papules
Physiologic hyperpigmentation
Plaque
Postinflammatory hyperpigmentation
Primary skin lesion
Pustule
Scales
Scar
Secondary skin lesion
Skene gland cyst
Syphilis
Trichomoniasis
Ulcer
Urethral caruncle
Urethral prolapse
Vesicle
Vestibular papillae
Wheal

References

Center for Disease Control and Prevention. (2010, December 17). Sexually transmitted diseases treatment guidelines. Retrieved January 1, 2010, from Center for Disease Control and Prevention: http://www.cdc.gov/std/treatment/2010/STD-Treatment-2010-RR5912.pdf

Edwards, L., & Lynch, P. (2010). *Genital dermatology atlas* (2nd ed.). Philadelphia: Lippincott, Williams & Wilkins.

Habif, T. (2009). *Clinical dermatology* (5th ed.). Philadelphia: Mosby.

Hainer, B. & Gibson, M. (2011). Vaginitis: Diagnosis and treatment. *American Family Physician (83)*8, 807–815.

Handsfield, H. (2001). *Color atlas & synopsis of sexually transmitted diseases* (2nd ed.). New York: McGraw-Hill.

Jarvis, C. (2008). *Physical examination & health assessment* (5th ed.). St. Louis, MO: Saunders.

Patton, K., & Thibodeau, G. (2010). *Anatomy and physiology* (7th ed.). St. Louis, MO: Mosby Elsevier.

Trott, A. (2005). *Wounds and lacerations: Emergency care and closure* (3rd ed.). Philadelphia: Mosby.

Weller, R., Hunter, J., Savin, J., & Dahl, M. (2008). *Clinical dermatology* (4th ed.). Malden, MA: Blackwell Publishing.

Wilkinson, E., & Stone, I. (2008). *Atlas of vulvar disease* (2nd ed.). Philadelphia: Lippincott Williams & Wilkins.

World Health Organization (WHO). (2011). *Sexually transmitted diseases*. Retrieved April 11, 2011, from http://www.who.int/vaccine_research/diseases/soa_std/en/index.html

CHAPTER 5

CONSENSUAL SEX INJURY

Jenifer Markowitz and Jennifer Pierce-Weeks

INTRODUCTION

Sexual contact, whether nonconsensual or consensual, can result in injury to the female genitalia, specifically when digital or penile penetration of the vagina occurs or is attempted.

Unfortunately, research is limited as to the nature and extent of injury that may occur with consensual sexual contact; much of what is posited on this subject stems from anecdotal evidence rather than clinical studies. However, what is clear is that the presence of genital injury is not exclusive to nonconsensual sexual contact. This chapter will examine existing literature related to injuries from consensual sex, discuss gaps in current scientific literature, and examine the clinical and legal importance of these consensual sexual contact injuries.

LITERATURE REVIEW

For decades, rates of anogenital injury found during medical evaluation following nonconsensual sex have varied widely.

More recent literature suggests injury rates ranging from 20% to 53% following sexual assault (Anderson, Parker, Bourguignon, 2009; Teerapong, Lumbiganon, Limpongsanurak, Udomprasertgul, 2009; White, McLean, 2006; Eckert, Sugar, Fine, 2004; Sugar, Fine, Eckert, 2004).

The use of the Masters and Johnson theory of **human sexual response** (1966) has been frequently employed to explain **genital injury** in patients after sexual assault. The theory holds that the normal physiologic changes that take place during consensual sexual activity, such as lubrication, lengthening of the vaginal outlet, and pelvic tilt, are protective in conjunction with mutual cooperation between sexual partners. Therefore, according to the theory, the presence of **anogenital injury** would be more likely in situations where the human sexual response did not occur, as in sexual assault. However, Masters and Johnson did not look at the presence or absence of injury in consensual sexual

activity. Additionally, recent studies documenting the presence of injury in consensual sex have shed significant doubt on the veracity of this theory.

The science is still emerging regarding the frequency and types of injury from consensual sexual contact, but the clinical picture has begun to take shape. See Table 5-1 for an overview of existing research specific to **consensual sex injury**.

Several studies have examined the prevalence of genital injury in patients presenting after consensual sex, with findings ranging from 5% to 73% (Lauber, Souma, 1982; Norvell, Benrubi, Thompson, 1984; Slaughter, Brown, Crowley, Peck, 1997; Jones, Rossman, Hartman, Alexander, 2003; Anderson, McClain, Riviello, 2006; McLean, Roberts, White, Paul, 2010; Sommers, Fargo, Baker, Fisher, 2009).

Note that there were discrepancies between the studies in the inclusion of **erythema** as a positive finding, which may account for some of the variation in prevalence data. Use of specialty techniques such as the **colposcope** and **toluidine blue dye** may also be a cause of variation; although, of the studies previously mentioned, examiners in only the McLean (2010) study (with consensual sex injuries identified in 6% of patients) failed to use either a colposcope or toluidine blue dye, instead relying solely upon direct visualization by the examiner.

Race and skin tone should also be considered when discussing prevalence of injury.

Sommers and colleagues (2008, 2009) identified consensual sex injury with greater frequency in white women than black woman (68% and 43%, respectively). Moreover, they found that white women were four times more likely to have one anogenital injury, and three times more likely to have two or more anogenital injuries than their black counterparts. Skin tone more than race was believed to be significant in the ability to identify injury.

Location of injuries was reviewed in several studies. Of significance is that none of the studies found posterior fourchette injury, particularly lacerations, to

TABLE 5-1 Overview of Existing Research on Consensual Sex Injury

Article	Study Overview	Findings
Comparison of methods for identifying anogenital injury after consensual intercourse. (2010) Zink T, Fargo JD, Baker RB, et al. J Emerg Med. 2010 Jul;39(1):113-118.	Comparison of consensual intercourse-related anogenital injury prevalence using 3 different forensic examination techniques: 1) direct visualization, 2) colposcopy, and 3) toluidine blue dye application. 120 woman ages 21 and older were examined following consensual sexual intercourse. The time between intercourse and examination ranged from 1 to 23 hours.	55% of patients who had consensual sex had injury. The use of toluidine blue dye resulted in a significantly higher prevalence of tears and abrasions on the external genitalia than when either direct visualization or colposcopy was used. Direct visualization and use of the colposcope were more effective at identifying contusions and redness.
Female genital injuries resulting from consensual and nonconsensual vaginal intercourse. (2011) McLean I, Roberts SA, White C, Paul S. Forensic Sci Int. May 28; 204(1–3), 27–33.	Two cohorts were recruited: a retrospective cohort of 500 sexual assault patients and 68 women recruited at the time of their routine cervical smear test who had recently had sexual intercourse.	Almost 23% of sexual assault patients sustained an injury to the genitalia, visible within 48 hours of the incident. This was 3 times more than the 5.9% of women who sustained a genital injury during consensual sex.
Changes in genital injury patterns over time in women after consensual intercourse. (2008) Anderson SL, Parker BJ, Bourguignon CM. J Forensic Leg Med. Jul;15(5):306-311.	Women (n = 35) ages 18-39 had two "evidentiary type" pelvic examinations to document injuries after consensual intercourse. 49% reported digital penetration of the vagina in addition to penile penetration of the vagina	At Time 1 (within 48 hours of consensual intercourse) there was a larger total surface area of injury, a larger surface area of injury to the posterior fourchette, a larger surface area of abrasions, and a larger surface area of redness compared to Time 2 (24 hours after Time 1).
Forensic sexual assault examination and genital injury: is skin color a source of health disparity? (2008) Sommers MS, Zink TM, Fargo JD, Baker RB, et al. Am J Emerg Med, 26, 857-866. Health disparities in the forensic sexual assault examination related to skin color. (2009) Sommers MS, Fargo JD, Baker RB, et al. J Forensic Nurs. 5(4):191-200.	This study compared anogenital injury prevalence and frequency in women of different races following consensual sexual intercourse. 120 women (63 black, 57 white) underwent a medical-forensic sexual assault examination following consensual sexual intercourse. Direct visualization, colposcopy with digital imaging, and toluidine blue dye were used to document the number, type, and location of anogenital injuries.	55% of the participants had at least one anogenital injury following consensual intercourse. Percentages differed significantly between white (68%) participants and black (43%) participants; however, percentage of injury was significantly different for injuries occurring only at the external genitalia (white, 56%; black, 24%), not for the internal genitalia (white, 28%; black, 19%), or anus (white, 9%; black, 10%). Dark skin color rather than race was a strong predictor for decreased injury prevalence.

Continued

TABLE 5-1 Overview of Existing Research on Consensual Sex Injury—cont'd

Article	Study Overview	Findings
Genital findings of women after consensual and nonconsensual intercourse. (2006) Anderson S, McClain N, Riviello RJ. J Forensic Nurs. 2(2):59-65.	102 women examined after consensual sex versus 56 following reported sexual assault.	No statistical difference was noted in the presence of injury between the 2 groups. The subjects in the nonconsensual group were 8 times more likely to have 2 or more injuries as the consensual group. There was a statistically significant difference in the injuries to the labia minora: only those in the nonconsensual group had injuries identified in this location.
Anogenital injuries in adolescents after consensual sexual intercourse. (2003) Jones JS, Rossman L, Hartman M, Alexander CC. Acad Emerg Med. Dec;10(12): 1378-1383.	51 adolescent females ages 13 to 17 were examined following reported consensual sex (49% for the first time); compared to control group of sexual assault patients.	Comparison of documented anogenital trauma: 73% of participants after consensual sex versus 85% of sexual assault patients. Consensual sex patients had injuries commonly involving hymen, fossa navicularis, and posterior fourchette. Patients who had nonconsensual sex had a greater number of injuries involving the fossa navicularis, labia minora, and hymen. The most common type of injury in both groups was lacerations. Sexual assault patients had more anogenital abrasions, bruising, and edema.
Variations in vaginal epithelial surface appearance determined by colposcopic inspection in healthy, sexually active women. (1999) Fraser IS, Lähteenmäki P, Elomaa K, et al. Hum Reprod. Aug;14(8):1974-1978.	107 women were examined 2-3 times over a 4- to 6-month period using a colposcope. Exams were meant to identify changes to the vaginal and cervical appearance caused by sexual intercourse, tampon use, contraception, and smoking or environmental factors.	In the 314 exams completed, the most common finding was petechiae. Actual lesions, defined primarily as tears, bruises or abrasions, occurred in only 3.5% of inspections, and were associated with sexual intercourse within the previous 24 hours or with tampon use.

TABLE 5-1 Overview of Existing Research on Consensual Sex Injury—cont'd		
Article	Study Overview	Findings
Patterns of genital injury in female sexual assault victims. (1997) Slaughter L, Brown CR, Crowley S, Peck R. Am J Obstet Gynecol. Mar;176(3): 609-616.	Physical examinations were performed on 311 rape victims seen by San Luis Obispo County's Suspected Abuse Response Team between 1985 and 1993 and contemporaneously on 75 women after consensual sexual intercourse.	Among 213 (68%) victims with genital trauma, 162 (76%) had approximately 3 mean sites of injury. 8 (11%) consenting women had just single-site trauma. 200 (94%) victims had trauma at 1 or more of 4 locations: posterior fourchette, labia minora, hymen, fossa navicularis. Trauma varied by site: tears on the posterior fourchette and fossa, abrasions on the labia, and bruising on the hymen.
Investigation of microtrauma after sexual intercourse. (1984) Norvell MK, Benrubi GI, Thompson RJ. J Reprod Med. Apr;29(4):269-271.	The study looked at whether a colposcope would help identify findings consistent with recent sexual intercourse. 18 participants were examined after 72 hours of abstinence and again 6 hours after sexual intercourse.	61% percent of patients had identifiable trauma following consensual sexual intercourse, compared to 11% following abstinence.
Use of toluidine blue dye for documentation of traumatic intercourse. (1982) Lauber AA, Souma ML. Obstet Gynecol. Nov;60(5): 644-648.	44 women were examined using toluidine blue dye, half of whom had had consensual sexual intercourse.	Only 1 of the 22 consensual sex patients had positive findings with toluidine blue dye, versus 40% of patients seen within 48 hours of sexual assault.

From Markowitz, J. (2010). *Consensual Sex Injury Clinical Guide.* Forensic Healthcare Online. Used with permission of the author.

be exclusive to nonconsensual sex. Jones, Rossman, Hartman, Alexander (2003) and Anderson, McClain, Riviello (2006) found injury to the **labia minora** to be more indicative of nonconsensual sexual intercourse than injuries to the **posterior fourchette**, hymen, or **fossa navicularis**. Other studies noted the presence of labia minora injury as a frequent occurrence in sexual assault patients (Slaughter, Brown, Crowley, Peck, 1997), but didn't provide comparison data for patients who were examined following consensual sex; or identified labia minora injury in consensual sex patients, but didn't detail the prevalence of said findings

(Anderson, Parker, Bourguignon, 2008). Furthermore, it is unclear whether there were commonalities regarding the mechanisms of injury (e.g., digital, penile, or foreign object penetration) in patients with injuries to specific sites. And only a few studies (Jones, Rossman, Hartman, Alexander, 2003; McLean, Roberts, White, Paul, 2010) looked at both location and types of injury in tandem with lacerations most commonly found on the posterior fourchette and fossa navicularis; abrasions on the labia minora; and bruising on the **cervix** and **hymen** (Figures 5-1 and 5-2).

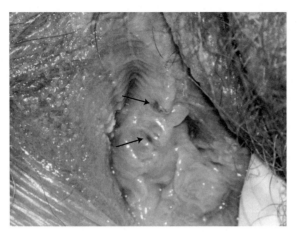

Figure 5-1
Bruising on hymen at the 9 o'clock and 11 o'clock positions.

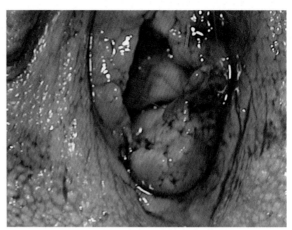

Figure 5-2
Bruising on hymen between the 2 o'clock and 4 o'clock positions; lacerations on hymen at the 3 o'clock and 7 o'clock positions.

Overall, **lacerations** were noted by several studies to be common injuries following consensual sexual intercourse as demonstrated in Figures 5-3 to 5-9 (McLean, Roberts, White, Paul, 2010; Jones, Rossman, Hartman, Alexander, 2003; Anderson, McClain, Riviello, 2006).

Bruising was often identified as a finding more common following nonconsensual sex.

Anderson and colleagues (2006) noted a fivefold increase in incidence of bruising and a fourfold increase in incidence of abrasions in nonconsensual sex subjects. Jones, Rossman, Hartman, and Alexander (2003) also found bruising to be more common in nonconsensual sex subjects. However, McLean, Roberts, White, and Paul (2010) actually identified bruising as the most common finding in the consensual sex subjects. Slaughter, Brown, Crowley, and Peck (1997) identified **hypervascularity** as the most common finding among patients following consensual sex and Frasier and colleagues (1999) identified **petechiae** and erythema as the most common findings in their study. Some of the

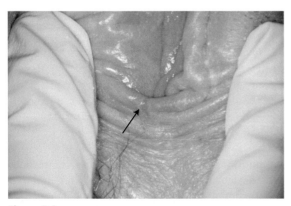

Figure 5-3
Laceration on posterior fourchette.

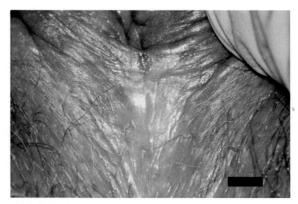

Figure 5-4
Laceration on posterior fourchette.

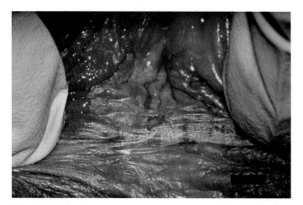

Figure 5-5
Laceration on posterior fourchette.

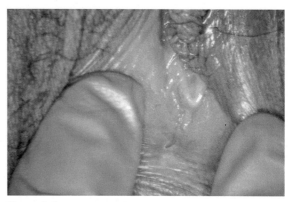

Figure 5-6
Laceration on fossa navicularis.

mechanisms of injury discussed were attributed to tampon use and speculum manipulation, not just to consensual sexual intercourse.

> Comparison studies of consensual and nonconsensual sex found that the number of injury sites appear to correlate with type of sexual intercourse, with greater numbers of injury appearing as a more common finding in nonconsensual sex subjects.

When two or more anogenital injuries were noted, Anderson and colleagues (2006) found that participants in their study were almost 10 times more likely to be in the nonconsensual sex group. McLean, Roberts, White, and Paul (2010) also

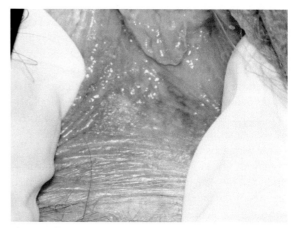

Figure 5-7
Laceration on fossa navicularis.

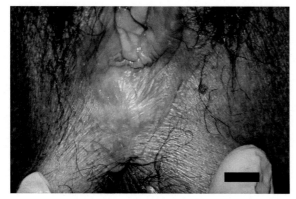

Figure 5-8
Laceration on perineum.

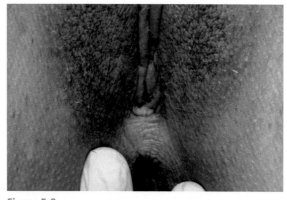

Figure 5-9
Lacerations on perineum and posterior fourchette.

identified multiple injuries more frequently in women examined following nonconsensual sex. Furthermore, Slaughter's study (1997) found that none of the women examined in the consensual sex group had more than one injury.

> The existing research regarding injury following consensual sex is fraught with limitations, so drawing firm conclusions is difficult.

Perhaps the greatest limitation, both in comparison studies of consensual and nonconsensual sex, and in stand-alone studies of consensual sex, is the small number of subjects studied. As mentioned before, the methods used to identify (the use of specialty techniques) and classify (the inclusion or exclusion of erythema) injury contribute to a broad disparity in injury prevalence in patients following consensual sex. Types of **vaginal penetration** are not always discussed in these studies, so it is difficult to know if consensual **digital penetration**, for instance, results in a similarly high frequency of injury as it does in nonconsensual sex (Rossman, et al, 2004).

The ways in which subjects were labeled in the studies may also be problematic. For instance, in the study conducted by Slaughter and colleagues (1997) the vast majority of the participants in the consensual sex comparison group actually presented as patients reporting sexual assault, but were later deemed to have cases that were unfounded. They were then moved to the consensual sex group; although, it is unclear whether any of the subjects had actually experienced consensual sexual contact. In the study by Frasier and colleagues (1999), it is unclear whether patients were ever screened for sexual violence, either prior to, or during the study period. Mention is made of "prolonged and intense intercourse" (p. 1976), but the possibility of nonconsensual sex does not appear to have been explored.

> The need for ongoing research on this subject is critical. Beyond the need for studies with greater sample sizes, there are several gaps in the research, including studies looking at consensual oral and anal sex, injuries in men, injuries among same-sex couples, and comparisons of length of healing time in consensual versus nonconsensual sex.

Examination of how these types of injuries manifest themselves in postmenopausal women is also greatly needed, along with research regarding injury differences among a broader ethnic and racial spectrum.

CLINICAL APPLICATION

Most clinicians who evaluate acute sexual assault victims do so in the emergency department (ED) or a sexual assault specific community-based health center. (Unpublished Data, IAFN, 2011). Rarely do patients present to the ED or sexual assault center with a complaint of genital injury following consensual sex. This limits the examiner's experiential understanding of genital injuries to those found following nonconsensual sex.

Clinicians typically evaluating patients who may have recently engaged in consensual sexual activity do so in primary care or public health settings. Typically it is an incidental finding that a patient had recently engaged in consensual sex rather than such activity as the primary complaint for which the patient is being seen (e.g. routine pap smear, mammogram). Additionally, when a patient is seen in the primary care setting the examination techniques differ slightly from those routinely employed during a sexual assault evaluation. For instance, in primary care examinations, specialty techniques such as toluidine blue dye application are not used, and more time is spent evaluating internal rather than external genital structures where injury is more likely to be observed.

> It is important that both clinicians and criminal justice system representatives understand that in any healthcare setting, the evaluation of a patient is largely driven by the history obtained from the patient.

If the patient is describing a sexual assault, the clinician should shift focus to ensure that the community-based standard of care for sexual assault medical-forensic examinations is met. If the patient is seeing her primary provider for a routine health check-up and, in the context of providing a health history, describes recent sexual intercourse, the approach is entirely different.

The knowledge of similarities and differences between injuries seen in consensual versus nonconsensual sexual activity has implications for clinicians who conduct sexual assault exams. Trained sexual assault examiners are often subpoenaed to testify about the care given to a specific sexual assault victim, particularly in the context of a prosecution. It is equally common that the examiner is qualified as an expert and asked to speak directly to the examination findings and her/his opinion regarding these findings. In criminal proceedings where consent is an issue, the clinician should expect to be asked if the injury seen could have been caused by consensual sexual activity or other possible causes of injury (e.g., disease process, hygiene issues).

> In this instance it is critical that the clinician have a fundamental understanding of the current medical literature on anogenital injury, including what is and is not known regarding injury following consensual sex.

Clinicians who care for patients presenting with the chief complaint of sexual assault need to be competent not only in the evaluation of anogenital injury, but in educating community partners (e.g., law enforcement, advocates, attorneys) regarding the presence or absence of injury and its meaning, as well as providing ethical testimony regarding how these injuries can be acquired.

It is important that clinicians participate in continuing education specific to the evaluation and assessment of sexual assault patients as a means to keep their practice current, and are able to analyze the body of literature related to anogenital injury and not rely on data culled from a single source.

> When called upon to provide an expert opinion, that opinion should be supported by the scientific literature and the clinician's own experience, not on anecdotes shared by other clinicians on listservs or via non-scientific Internet resources (e.g., Wikipedia).

Key Terms

Anogenital injury
Bruise
Cervix
Colposcope
Consensual sex injury
Digital penetration
Erythema
Fossa navicularis
Genital injury
Human sexual response
Hymen
Hypervascularity
Labia minora
Laceration
Petechiae
Posterior Fourchette
Race
Toluidine blue dye
Vaginal penetration

References

Anderson, S., McClain, N., & Riviello, R. J. (2006). Genital findings of women after consensual and nonconsensual intercourse. *Journal of Forensic Nursing, 2*(2), 59–65.

Anderson, S. L., Parker, B. J., & Bourguignon, C. M. (2008). Changes in genital injury patterns over time in women after consensual intercourse. *Journal of Forensic and Legal Medicine, 15*(5), 306–311.

Anderson, S. L., Parker, B. J., & Bourguignon, C. M. (2009). Predictors of genital injury after nonconsensual intercourse. *Advanced Emergency Nursing Journal, 31*(3), 236–247.

Eckert, L. O., Sugar, N., & Fine, D. (2004). Factors impacting injury documentation after sexual assault: Role of examiner experience and gender. *American Journal of Obstetrics and Gynecology, 190*(6), 1739–1743, discussion 1744–1746.

Forensic Healthcare Online. (2010). *Consensual Sex Injury Clinical Guide.* Retrieved from http://www.forensichealth.com/2010/09/21/consensual-sex-injury/

Fraser, I. S., Lähteenmäki, P., Elomaa, K., et al. (1999). Variations in vaginal epithelial surface appearance determined by colposcopic inspection in healthy, sexually active women. *Human Reproduction, 14*(8), 1974–1978.

International Association of Forensic Nurses. [Unpublished data]. Retrieved May 26, 2011.

Jones, J. S., Rossman, L., Hartman, M., & Alexander, C. C. (2003). Anogenital injuries in adolescents after consensual sexual intercourse. *Academic Emergency Medicine, 10*(12), 1378–1383.

Lauber, A. A., & Souma, M. L. (1982). Use of toluidine blue for documentation of traumatic intercourse. *Obstetrics and Gynecology, 60*(5), 644–648.

Masters, W. H., & Johnson, V. E. (1966). *Human sexual response.* (1st ed.). Boston: Little, Brown.

McLean, I., Roberts, S. A., White, C., & Paul, S. (2011). Female genital injuries resulting from consensual and nonconsensual intercourse. *Forensic Science International, 204*(1–3), 27–33.

Norvell, M. K., Benrubi, G. I., & Thompson, R. J. (1984). Investigation of microtrauma after sexual intercourse. *Journal of Reproductive Medicine, 29*(4), 269–271.

Rossman, L., Jones, J. S., Dunnuck, C., et al. (2004). Genital trauma associated with forced digital penetration. *American Journal of Emergency Medicine, 22*(2), 101–104.

Slaughter, L., Brown, C. R., Crowley, S., & Peck, R. (1997). Patterns of genital injury in female sexual assault victims. *American Journal of Obstetrics and Gynecology, 176*(3), 609–616.

Sommers, M. S., Fargo, J. D., Baker, R. B., et al. (2009). Health disparities in the forensic sexual assault examination related to skin color. *Journal of Forensic Nursing 5*(4), 191–200.

Sommers, M. S., Zink, T. M., Fargo, J. D., et al. (2008). Forensic sexual assault examination and genital injury: Is skin color a source of health disparity? *American Journal of Emergency Medicine, 26*, 857–866.

Sugar, N. F., Fine, D. N., & Eckert, L. O. (2004). Physical injury after sexual assault: Findings of a large case series. *American Journal of Obstetrics and Gynecology, 190*(1), 71–76.

Teerapong, S., Lumbiganon, P., Limpongsanurak, S., & Udomprasertgul, V. (2009). Physical health consequences of sexual assault victims. *Journal of the Medical Association of Thailand, 92*(7), 885–890.

White, C., & McLean, I. (2006). Adolescent complainants of sexual assault; injury patterns in virgin and non-virgin groups. *Journal of Clinical Forensic Medicine, 13*(4), 172–180.

Zink, T., Fargo, J. D., Baker, R. B., et al. (2010). Comparison of methods for identifying ano-genital injury after consensual intercourse. *The Journal of Emergency Medicine, 39*(1), 113–118.

CHAPTER 6

ANOGENITAL INJURY

Linda Rossman, Jeffrey Jones, and Christine K. Dunnuck

Since the mid-1980s, a number of studies have examined the incidence of anogenital trauma in female sexual assault victims. **Anogenital** injuries from consensual and nonconsensual sexual intercourse range from rapidly healing superficial lacerations to major vault and mucosal lacerations. Some researchers have reported rates of anogenital injuries of only 5% to 28% among sexual assault cases; others have suggested that rates are higher now that trauma can be detected using stain and magnification procedures (Biggs, Stermac, Divinsky, 1998; Sachs, Chu, 2002). It may be impossible to determine true injury incidence and patterns because so many cases go unreported to law enforcement or healthcare providers. As a result, study samples are limited to include only those individuals who present to healthcare settings stating they are a victim of sexual assault.

> Many variables are not fully understood in how they might influence sexual assault-related physical trauma (Gaffney, 2003).

These variables can be grouped in the following manner: factors related to the victim (e.g., age, ethnicity, hormonal status, previous sexual experience); the assailant (e.g., object of penetration, gang versus individual, relationship to victim); the circumstances (e.g., coercion, weapons, alcohol or drug use); and the environment (i.e., location).

> Whether a person having **consensual** or **nonconsensual sex** will suffer genital injuries, and under what conditions, remains difficult to predict.

This chapter will review the literature as it relates to injury prevalence, location, and documentation. Forensic techniques to aid the examiner in the medical-forensic examination will also be discussed.

INJURY PREVALENCE

Prevalence and incidence of anogenital injury in reported sexual assaults are often the focus of healthcare research. **Prevalence** of injury is defined as the total number of injuries at a given time within a population of those reporting sexual assault. **Incidence** indicates a measure of risk of sustaining injury during sexual assault. Presentation of physical findings in sexual assault can range from no injuries to severe life-threatening ones. Most injuries related to sexual assault are minor. Moderate to severe trauma has been reported in up to 18% of victims; however, less than 1% of those required hospitalization (Alempijevic, Savic, Plavekic, Jecmenica, 2006; Slaughter, Brown, Crowley, Peck, 1997). It is unknown how many victims required additional medical care prior to discharge as an outpatient. Although proof of resistance is no longer a legal requirement, the public, including many judges and juries, still perceive injury, especially genital injury, as the essential proof that the victim did not consent to intercourse (Gaffney, 2003).

> There are several reasons why victims may not exhibit evidence of anogenital trauma upon examination. The anatomy of the reproductive structures, type of penetration, and the health and age of the victim may contribute to the absence of anogenital injury. Weapons or threat of injury may intimidate victims into complying with the offender, or alcohol and/or drugs ingested can render victims physically incapable of resisting an assault. Many women are reluctant to seek treatment immediately following an assault and may wait several hours or days before seeking medical care.

Anogenital injuries are seen more frequently in patients who are examined within 24 hours after the assault, as well as in those who are subjected to anal assault (Sugar, Fine, Eckert, 2004).

The prevalence of anogenital injury after sexual assault ranges in the literature from 5% (Massey, Garcia, Emich, 1971) to 87% (Slaughter, Brown, 1992). Differences in findings can be attributed to different examination techniques used in these studies, including direct visualization, colposcopic magnification, and staining techniques. Colposcopic technique with digital image or photographic capture is routinely used in sexual assault medical-forensic examinations in the United States (U.S. Department of Justice, 2004). Colposcope use has been associated with the documentation of a higher prevalence of injury than other techniques, particularly when combined with staining preparations such as toluidine blue dye (Sommers, 2007).

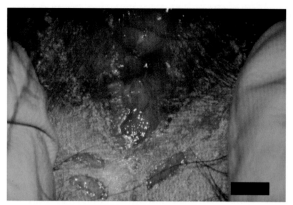

Figure 6-1
   Posterior fourchette and perineum lacerations.

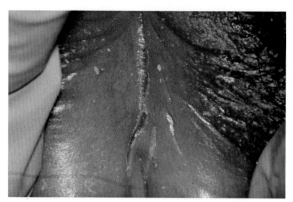

Figure 6-2
   Labia minora laceration midline at the 12 o'clock position.

Use of some visualization adjunct is important because many anogenital injuries are subtle and may be difficult to detect by examiners who do not regularly assess sexually assaulted patients. To date there has been no pattern of injury or constellation of findings that can verify with any statistical significance the occurance of sexual assault.

INJURY LOCATION

The most common locations for genital injury in female **adolescent**s and women are the **posterior fourchette** (Figure 6-1), **labia minora** (Figures 6-2 and 6-3), **hymen** (Figures 6-4 to 6-6), and **fossa navicularis** (Figure 6-7) (Grossin, Sibille, Lorin de la Gradmaison, et al., 2003; Jones, Rossman, Wynn, et al., 2003; Lauber, Souma, 1982; Slaughter, Brown, 1992; Slaughter, Brown, Crowley, Peck, 1997; Sommers, Schafer, Zink, et al., 2001).

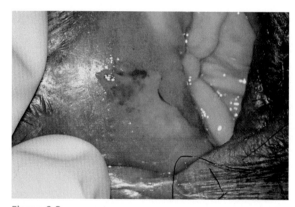

Figure 6-3
   Right labia minor abrasion between the 7 o'clock and 8 o'clock positions.

Of those with genital injury, Slaughter and colleagues (1997) found genital injury most often at the posterior forchette (70%), labia minora (53%), hymen (29%), and fossa navicularis (25%). Most women report being sexually assaulted in a supine position and common sites of injury are to the fossa navicularis and posterior fourchette in the 5 o'clock and 7 o'clock positions. This may be because the posterior fourchette and fossa navicularis are generally the first structures of the genitalia that come in contact with an erect penis during penile vaginal

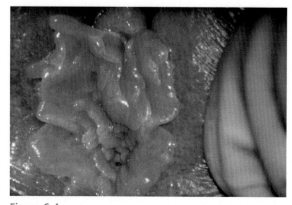

Figure 6-4
   Swelling of hymenal edges.

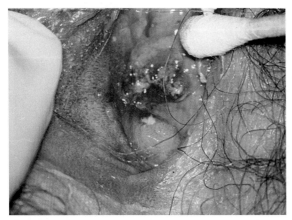

Figure 6-5
Hymen laceration with bruising at the 8 o'clock and 9 o'clock positions.

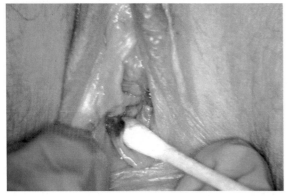

Figure 6-6
Hymen laceration with bruising at the 3 o'clock and 8 o'clock positions.

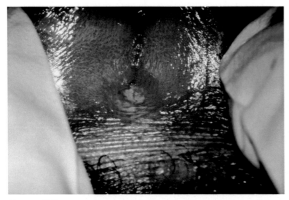

Figure 6-7
Fossa navicularis laceration.

penetration (Rosay, Henry, 2008). Jones, Rossman, Wynn, and colleagues (2003) reported similar findings in 766 women and pubertal girls younger than age 18. They found 78% had injuries at one of the four locations mentioned, although adult women experienced less injury to the hymen and greater injury to the perianal area compared with adolescent pubertal females. Although the posterior fourchette, labia minora, hymen, and fossa navicularis are the most common sites of injury seen in sexual assault victims, injuries do occur on the **mons pubis** (Figure 6-8), **labia majora** (Figures 6-9 and 6-10), labia majora/minora junction (Figure 6-11), **clitoral hood** (Figure 6-12), **perineum** (Figure 6-13), **vaginal walls** (Figures 6-14 and 6-15), **cervix** (Figure 6-16), **anus** (Figures 6-17 and 6-18), **anal canal** (Figures 6-19 and 6-20), and **rectum** (Figures 6-21 and 6-22); therefore,

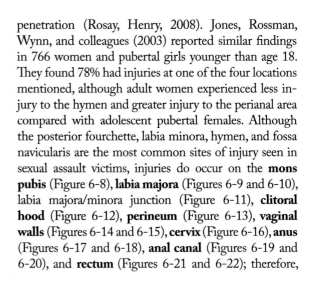

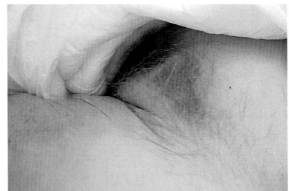

Figure 6-8
Mons pubis bruising.

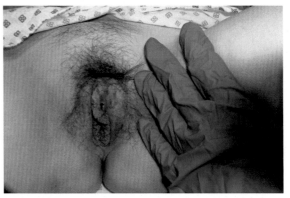

Figure 6-9
Left labium majus bruising from the 1 o'clock to the 5 o'clock positions. Left labia minor bruising from the 1 o'clock to the 3 o'clock positions.

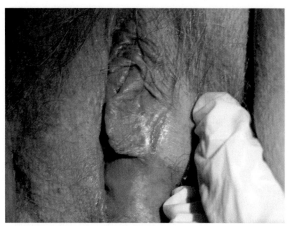

Figure 6-10
Left labium majus laceration from the 3 o'clock to the 4 o'clock positions.

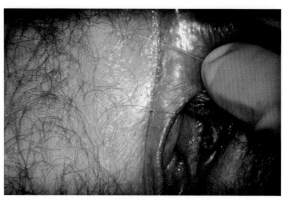

Figure 6-11
Right labia major/minor junction laceration from the 7 o'clock to the 11 o'clock positions.

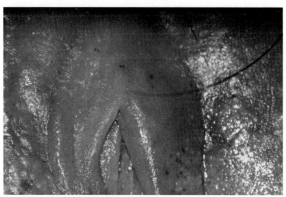

Figure 6-12
Clitoral hood petechiae from the 10 o'clock to the 2 o'clock positions. Patient reported forced cunnilingus during sexual assault.

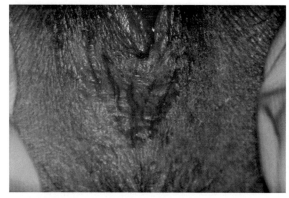

Figure 6-13
Multiple lacerations on perineum.

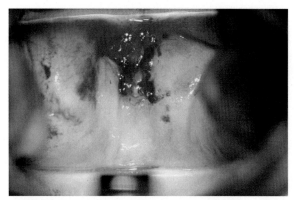

Figure 6-14
Vaginal cuff laceration with bruising and frank bleeding. Note atrophic postmenopausal tissue and lack of cervix from hysterectomy.

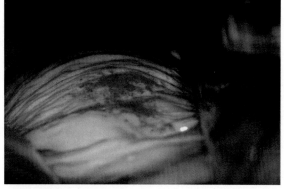

Figure 6-15
Posterior vaginal wall bruising.

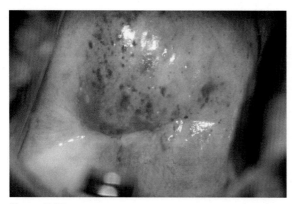

Figure 6-16
Cervical bruising and petechiae.

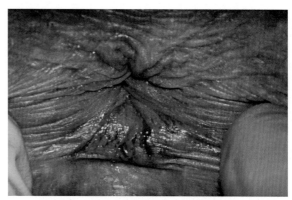

Figure 6-17
Multiple anal lacerations from the 5 o'clock to the 7 o'clock positions.

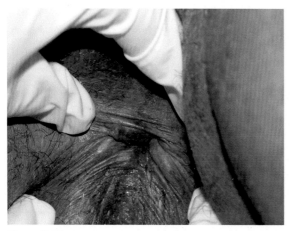

Figure 6-18
Anal lacerations at the 5 o'clock position.

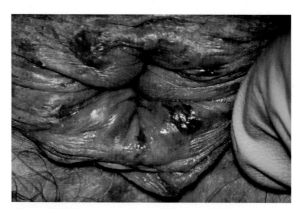

Figure 6-19
Anal canal abrasions at the 2 o'clock, 5 o'clock, 8 o'clock, and 10 o'clock positions. Laceration at the 6 o'clock position.

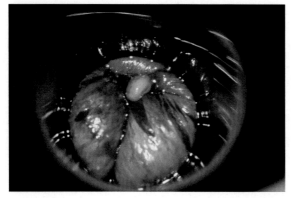

Figure 6-20
Anal canal lacerations at the 4 o'clock and 5 o'clock positions.

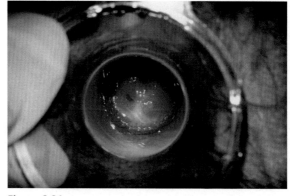

Figure 6-21
Rectal laceration at the 9 o'clock position with fresh bleeding.

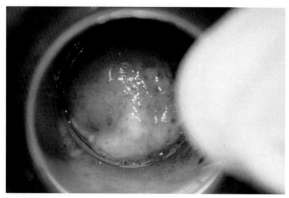

Figure 6-22
Rectal bruising.

examiners should closely inspect each anatomical site for injury in every examination.

INJURY DOCUMENTATION

Detailed documentation of anogenital injury should include the history and mechanism of the assault. This is necessary to provide comprehensive healthcare and to alert healthcare providers to possible occult injury, prompting consideration for emergency medical care or consultation and referral.

Information regarding the mechanism used in the assault will also help assist in determining risk exposure to sexually transmitted infections.

A critical point of consideration is that while identified injuries may corroborate victims' accounts, the absence of such injuries does not negate the possibility that a sexual assault took place.

In addition, two victims with similar assault history may not share the same physical injuries (Gaffney, 2003).

When documenting injuries, it is important to include size, location, and a detailed description of injuries. It is equally important to document pain or discomfort the patient may be experiencing during the examination. Use of a **pain scale** is appropriate and widely used by healthcare providers to assess a person's level of pain. One common scale is the 0 to 10 pain scale with 0 being no pain and 10 the worst pain a person has experienced.

COLPOSCOPIC EXAMINATION

Three primary techniques are used in the anogenital examination: colposcopy, staining, and direct visualization. Colposcopy is a procedure that allows a healthcare provider to perform a magnified visual inspection of the external and internal genitalia in the context of a standard gynecologic exam. It allows the user to identify and photograph bruising, abrasions, and lacerations that may occur during a sexual assault. As part of San Luis Obispo County's suspected abuse response team, Slaughter and Brown (1992) were the first to report the regular use of a colposcope for sexual assault examinations in adult women. They found that 87% of victims (N=131) had identifiable injury via colposcopic examination. Several years later, in a small prospective study, Lenahan, Ernst, and Johnson (1998) found that the colposcope allowed documentation of trauma in 9 of the 17 sexual assault victims (53%), compared with 1 of 17 (6%) by direct visualization alone.

Despite the lack of rigorous scientific evidence, the use of a colposcope in pediatric and adult sexual assault cases has become increasingly more widespread nationally.

A **colposcope** is now used to view anogenital or non-genital injuries in many sexual assault programs, emergency departments, and child advocacy centers.

Potential drawbacks to the routine use of a colposcope include the expense of purchasing and maintaining equipment, plus the additional provider training required to use the equipment efficiently. The first large-scale prospective clinical study to directly compare the three primary techniques for performing a medical-forensic sexual assault examination was recently published (Rogers, McIntyre, Rossman, Jones, 2008). Four hundred and forty-five cases of sexual assault were included in the study. Sixty-three percent of the anogenital injuries were identified with direct visualization alone. Additional lacerations and abrasions (34%) were identified with toluidine blue dye. Colposcopic examination identified only 3% more injuries than were already seen using direct visualization and toluidine blue dye staining. These injuries were typically localized **erythema** or edema involving the cervix, anal folds, and vagina. Overall, four women had subtle genital injuries detected only by colposcopic visualization. The authors concluded that when compared with direct visualization and nuclear staining, colposcopic visualization offered little advantage to a skilled, experienced forensic examiner. However, documenting injury rates and the ability to identify injuries can vary upon the visualization adjuncts, and more research in this area is needed.

TOLUIDINE BLUE DYE

> **Lacerations** to the posterior fourchette, fossa navicularis, labia majora, labia minora, and perineum might not be obvious by direct visualization, particularly for inexperienced examiners.

Toluidine blue dye is a nuclear stain commonly used to detect and document genital and **perianal** injuries. In early studies, application of a 1% solution of toluidine

blue dye increased the detection rate of posterior fourchette lacerations from 16% to 40% in adult sexual assault victims (Lauber, Souma, 1982; McCauley, Guzinski, Welch, et al., 1987).

If used to assist with visualization during the anogenital examination, toluidine blue dye should be applied to the posterior fourchette, fossa navicularis, labia minora, perineum, or anus prior to the insertion of the examiner's finger, speculum, or anoscope. Removal of the toluidine blue dye is completed by gently wiping the application site with gauze moistened with lubricating jelly or a 1% acetic acid solution. A negative result is indicated by either no uptake or light, diffusely stippled uptake of dye. A diffuse or stippled uptake is considered negative as this may be due to other causes, such as inflammation resulting from infection or vulvovaginal disease. A positive result is indicated by distinct deep, royal blue staining in skin defects (Figures 6-23 and 6-24).

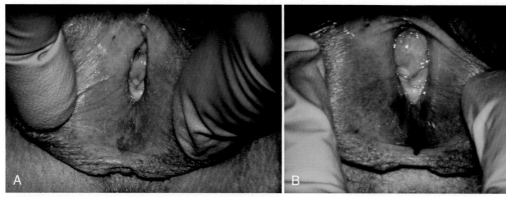

Figure 6-23
A, Fossa navicularis laceration before toluidine blue dye application. B, Fossa navicularis laceration after toluidine blue dye application.

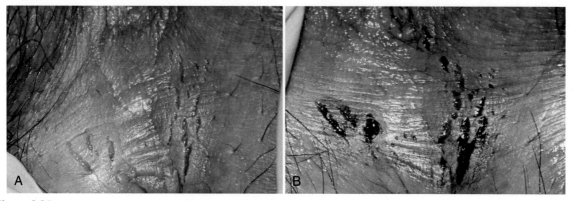

Figure 6-24
A, Multiple perineum lacerations before toluidine blue dye application. B, Multiple perineum lacerations after toluidine blue dye application.

Causes of positive uptake other than injury, such as fissures resulting from constipation, surgical procedures, or tampons must be considered as well.

FOLEY CATHETER TECHNIQUE

Estrogenized adolescent female hymens are often redundant, characterized by abundant tissue folded over itself with an irregular configuration (Starling, Jenny, 1997). These hymenal folds can mask areas of trauma.

> The **Foley catheter technique** is a simple, inexpensive method that allows improved visualization and photodocumentation of the estrogenized hymen in adolescents (Jones, Genco, Dunnuck, et al., 2003).

A 14 French Foley catheter is inserted through the hymenal orifice until the balloon is estimated to be midway in the vagina. The balloon is then inflated with 15 to 30 mL of air. Water is not used because it decreases buoyancy of the balloon and decreases visualization of the posterior hymen. The index finger may be used to guide the balloon to the hymen edge, while pulling gently on the Foley catheter with the other hand. The hymen is then expanded to its full capacity, and the edge of the hymen may be examined and photographed for the presence or absence of trauma (Figures 6-25 and 6-26).

The Foley catheter technique requires some manual dexterity to maintain labial traction while keeping gentle traction on the tubing and taking adequate photographs (Persaud, Squires, Rubin-Remer, 1997). This technique is useful in defining and photodocumenting acute injuries of the hymen. Other clinical

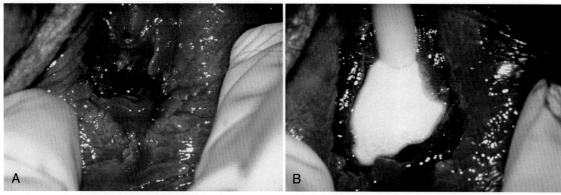

Figure 6-25
A, Hymen bruising and lacerations before Foley catheter technique. B, Hymen bruising and lacerations with Foley catheter technique.

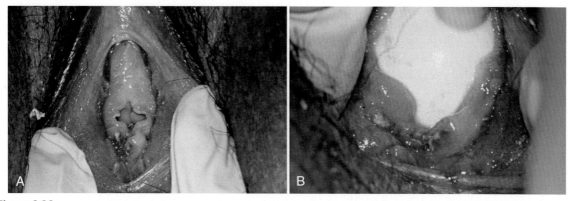

Figure 6-26
A, Hymen bruising and laceration before Foley catheter technique. B, Hymen bruising and laceration with Foley catheter technique.

findings such as partial clefts, hymenal notches, edema, erythema, and the width of the hymen potentially could be altered by the inflated balloon. Interpretations of nonspecific clinical findings using this technique must be made with care.

MALE SEXUAL ASSAULT VICTIMS

The majority of sexual assault literature focuses on women. Those studies that examined males as sexual assault victims have primarily examined the psychosocial aspects of sexual assault and most of the literature has been focused on the male pediatric population. Few studies have examined adolescent-adult male sexual assault victims and physical findings for the male. Saltzman and colleagues (2007) studied sexual violence treated in the emergency department and found men and boys make up nearly 11% of patients treated for sexual assault in emergency departments. Walker, Archer, and Davies (2005) found that men who seek treatment following sexual assault tend to do so long after the sexual assault has occurred and are more likely to seek treatment only if they are severely injured (Figures 6-27 to 6-29).

This same study concluded that men perceive they will be disbelieved, blamed, or treated negatively. These barriers, or perceived barriers, may contribute to the male sexual assault victim's decision to not report or seek treatment following an assault.

Masho and Alvanso (2009) studied health-seeking behaviors of men following sexual assault and found those who were threatened during the assault were seven and a half times more likely to seek professional care. They also found those who sustained physical injuries were eleven times more likely to seek help, and those assaulted by family or a friend were six times more likely to seek care.

Stermac, Del Bove, and Addison (2004) studied victim and assault characteristics among adult male victims in an urban emergency department sexual assault care center. They found that sexual assault of males more likely involved **fellatio** (see Figure 6-29) and anal assault compared with female victims. The assailant was typically male (93% to 97%). Weapon use and

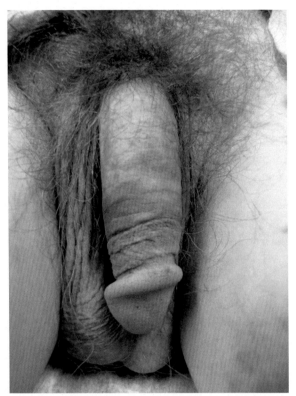

Figure 6-27
Penile shaft bruising.

multiple assailants were significantly higher in stranger rape than in acquaintance rape. The most common areas for anogenital injuries were the perineal and anal areas. These findings support earlier research by Lacey and Roberts (1991). As in females, the anogenital structures most injured are the point of initial contact, resulting in the tissue being stretched beyond its capacity to compensate, causing injury. Stermac and colleagues (2004) found the most common types of injury were soft tissue, including **bruises** and lacerations, and there were no significant difference in these findings between female and male sexual assault patients.

ADOLESCENT SEXUAL ASSAULT VICTIMS

One third of all victims of sexual assault who report to law enforcement agencies are adolescents between the ages of 13 to 17 years (Snyder, 2000). Adolescents and young adults are four times more likely to be victims

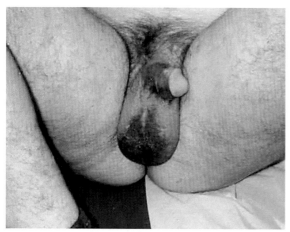

Figure 6-28
Penile and scrotal bruising. Scrotal laceration at the 6 o'clock position.

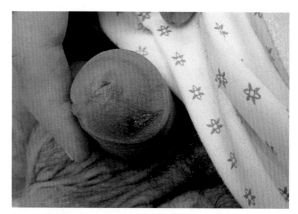

Figure 6-29
Periurethral bruising. Healing abrasion on the glans at the 3 o'clock position.

of sexual assault than women in all other age groups (Snyder 2000; Poirier, 2002). The epidemiology of sexual trauma and the patterns of anogenital trauma in this age group are unique and may pose special challenges to examiners. For example, the majority of adolescent sexual assaults are perpetrated by an acquaintance or relative of the adolescent. Using the expanded definition of incest, the U.S. Bureau of Justice Statistics reports 24% of rape victims between the ages of 12 to 17 years were attacked by a family member (Snyder, 2000).

Adolescent sexual assaults are less likely to involve weapons or physical coercion and are associated with fewer non-genital injuries (Adams, Girardin, Faugno, 2001). Adolescents have a greater frequency of anogenital injuries (83% versus 64%) when compared with older women (Jones, Rossman, Wynn, et al., 2003). It is important that the examiner is aware of the increased frequency of anogenital injuries in adolescents since they often are examined at programs housed in settings that predominantly serve adult patient populations (Baker, Sommers, 2008).

The recognition of abnormal physical findings in an adolescent victim of sexual assault must be based on an understanding of normal findings. The victim's age, stage of sexual development, state of relaxation, and methods used during the examination all contribute to the variable appearance of this anatomy (Chadwick, Berkowitz, Kerns, et al., 1989).

> Knowledge of the changes that occur naturally in the genitalia and perianal tissues as the adolescent matures is important for proper interpretation of physical findings.

Although some examiners may focus on hymenal tears when looking for genital trauma in adolescent sexual assault victims, the fossa navicularis is the most common site of injury in this population (Adams, Girardin, Faugno, 2001; Jones, Genco, Dunnuck, et al., 2003). Other vulnerable sites include the hymen, labia minora, and posterior fourchette (Figure 6-30). The injuries show consistent topologic features, varying with the site and nature of tissue. This pattern provides evidence that the major cause of genital trauma seen in adolescent sexual assault victims may be upon entry into the vagina with insertion or attempts at insertion of the penis (or finger or other object) (Slaughter, Brown, Crowley, Peck, 1997). The relative fixation of the posterior portion of the introitus to the perineal body, with its multiple muscular attachments, may account for a focusing of stresses and consequent tears in this region (Geist, 1988). Adult victims of sexual assault have a less consistent pattern of anogenital injuries owing to less documented hymenal trauma, greater injury to the perianal area, and widespread erythema. However, early research on patterns of injury suggest that some findings are more typical in nonconsensual intercourse, such as bruising of the labia in both adults

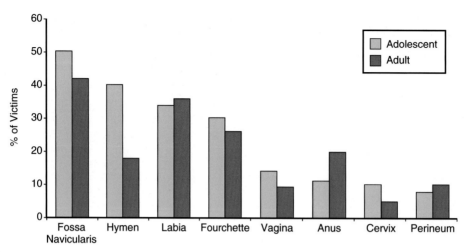

Figure 6-30

Location of injury in adolescent and adult sexual assault victims with anogenital findings. (From Jones, J. S., Rossman, L., Wynn, B., et al. (2003). Comparative analysis of adult versus adolescent sexual assault: Epidemiology and patterns of anogenital injury. *Academic Emergency Medicine, 10*(8), 872–877. Used with permission of the authors.)

(Anderson, McClain, Riviello, 2006) and adolescents (Jones, Rossman, Hartman, Alexander, 2004).

SEXUAL ASSAULT IN POSTMENOPAUSAL WOMEN

Physical abuse of older adults, including reports of sexual assault, has risen rapidly in the last decade (Burgess, Hanrahan, Baker, 2005). The true extent of this problem is difficult to determine. Reluctance to report sexual abuse, relative isolation of elderly victims, and lack of public and professional awareness undoubtedly contribute to many cases of undetected assault. In addition, sexual assault committed against women older than 50 years of age has been the subject of only scattered and limited scientific study. The National Crime Victimization Survey estimates the incidence of sexual assault committed against older adults at 50 per 100,000 per year, representing about 3% of all sexual assault victims in the United States (Sedgwick, 2006).

> Older sexual assault victims may be particularly susceptible to physical injury because of declining health and strength, decreased levels of estrogen, comorbidity, cognitive impairments, and psychopathologic condition of the offender (Del Bove, Stermac, Bainbridge, 2005).

Assaults on older women tend to be more violent and brutal than assaults on younger women. This higher level of violence is usually inflicted by an unknown assailant who forcibly enters the victim's home (Jones, Rossman, Diegel, et al., 2009).

A cohort analysis of 1,917 adult sexual assault victims reported **postmenopausal** women had a greater mean number of non-genital (2.3 versus 1.2) as well as anogenital (2.5 versus 1.8) injuries. The localized pattern and type of physical injuries were similar in both groups, although postmenopausal women tended to have more anogenital lacerations and abrasions (Jones, Rossman, Diegel, et al., 2009). The overall prevalence of anogenital injury was 64%. Most of the genital injuries (80%) occurred at 1 of 3 anatomical sites as follows: labia minora, fossa navicularis, and posterior fourchette.

It is also important to recognize that less serious injuries may have more serious consequences in morbidity and mortality among older adult patients. Schwab and Kauder (1992) report outcome differences between older and younger trauma patients are most disparate at the lower end of the injury scale. Thus, it is seemingly insignificant injuries that may need increased attention. Evidence of bruising to the perineum, pain with micturation, vaginal bleeding, and discharge are all warning signs (Feldhaus, Houry, Kaminsky, 2000). In addition to physical trauma, postmenopausal women may experience psychologic trauma that may be no less severe than in younger women, such as post-traumatic stress disorder and rape-trauma syndrome, for years after the assault.

SKIN PIGMENTATION AND CLINICAL FINDINGS

A review of the medical literature over the past few decades demonstrates subtle indications that racial and/or ethnic differences may be present in the prevalence of genital injury resulting from sexual assault. For example, Cartwright and the Sexual Assault Study Group (1987) found in a retrospective review of medical records that white women of all ages had genital injuries twice as frequently as black women. Coker, Walls, and Johnson (1998) studied male and female sexual assault victims and found among males that race (especially white) was significantly associated with traumatic physical injury when adjusting for other correlates. Among women, injury was not significantly associated with race. Sommers and colleagues (2006) found significant association between race (black versus white) and genital injury, indicating whites were more than four times as likely as blacks to have genital injury.

The majority of sexual assault research has been conducted with young white women, masking the distinct differences in predictors of injury in diverse racial groups in different regions of the United States. African-Americans and other racial groups may be less likely to report to police or be seen by healthcare providers after sexual assault due to societal and institutional mistrust (Clay-Warner, 2002). A recent study by Stevens, Jones, Rossman, and Wynn (2009) suggested individuals with darker skin may be at a disadvantage for injury identification with current examination strategies (direct visualization, nuclear staining, or colposcopic), and color awareness may be an important component of the sexual assault medical-forensic examination.

Although **skin pigmentation** is a socially charged issue, further research will be needed to understand racial and ethnic differences in genital injury prevalence and to explore mechanisms to control for skin pigmentation during the sexual assault examination.

DIGITAL OR FOREIGN BODY PENETRATION

Penetration of the vagina, anus, or oral cavity can occur with the penis, foreign objects, or fingers. An important role for the forensic examiner in cases of sexual assault is to document physical findings. However, when forced **digital penetration** is the only complaint, a medical–legal examination is often not performed (Geist, 1988). In a study of female sexual assault victims (Slaughter, Brown, Crowley, Peck, 1997) investigators found that digital penetration occurred in 43% of adult victims with positive anogenital injuries. In 2004, Rossman and colleagues published a study that examined genital trauma in women in whom forced digital penetration was the only allegation. Forced digital penetration is defined as any nonconsensual manipulation, fondling, or penetration of the vulvar area by the assailant's fingers. Genital injuries were documented in 81% of these patients. Fifty-six percent of the injuries occurred at four sites: fossa navicularis, labia minora, cervix, and posterior fourchette. The most common type of injury was erythema followed by lacerations and abrasions. Lacerations appeared most often on the posterior fourchette and fossa navicularis, abrasions appeared on the labia minora, and bruising was seen on the cervix and hymen. See Figures 6-31 to 6-33 for examples of injuries caused by digital penetration.

Foreign object penetration of the anogenitalia during a sexual assault can result in serious, sometimes fatal, injuries. Several case reports of such incidents have been reported (Delacroix, Brown, Kadenhe-Chiweshe, et al., 2011; Carey, Healy, Elder, 2010; Henry, 2010; Orr, Clark, Hawley, et al., 1995; Fain, McCormick, 1989); however, few studies have been published regarding anogenital findings identified in sexual assaults with foreign object penetration. A recent study by Sturgiss, Tyson, and Parekh (2010) found genital injuries were more likely to be documented when a foreign object was involved. They found 75% had genital injuries with foreign object penetration compared with 38% without. More research focusing on foreign object penetration should be done to gain a better understanding of the types, sites, and patterns of anogenital injury sustained in these types of assaults. See Figures 6-34 to 6-38 for examples of injuries caused by foreign objects.

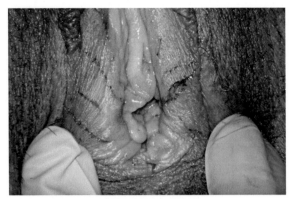

Figure 6-31
Lacerations on labia minora and posterior fourchette after digital penetration with 4 fingers simultaneously.

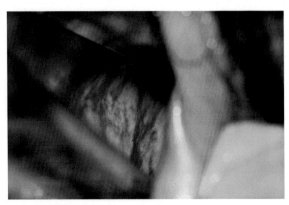

Figure 6-32
Abrasion and bruising on left lateral vaginal wall after digital penetration.

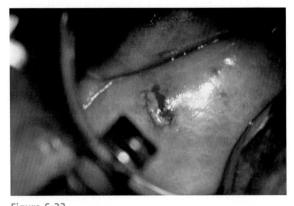

Figure 6-33
Cervical laceration with bleeding after digital penetration.

PRIOR SEXUAL INTERCOURSE

Whether a person having consensual or nonconsensual sex will suffer genital injuries, and under what conditions, remains difficult to predict.

Common knowledge and findings from studies of first consensual intercourse predict women who had no prior sexual intercourse experience (i.e., virgins) at the time of the assault would suffer more serious genital injuries. However, clinical evidence indicates not all cases of penetration result in subsequent visible genital injuries. Biggs, Stermac, Divinsky (1998) found that visible genital injuries occurred more frequently in women who had no prior sexual intercourse experience than in those who had (65% versus 26%). However, of the women without prior experience, only 9% had hymenal injury. Of women with genital injuries, data analysis suggested no significant statistical difference between those without prior sexual intercourse and those with prior sexual intercourse in the overall mean number of injured sites (1.65 and 1.47, respectively). The authors concluded substantial proportions of all women, regardless of their prior sexual experience at the time of assault, will not have visible genital injuries. This finding has been reported elsewhere (Rossman, Jones, Nelson-Horan, et al., 2000).

Whether an adolescent female has had prior sexual intercourse is impossible to determine from examining the genitalia.

Because of the effects of estrogen, the adolescent hymen is elastic and can permit penile penetration without tearing. In addition, genitourinary trauma can heal rapidly so even small hymenal lacerations are not present several days after an assault (Poirier, 2002). Slaughter and colleagues (1997) reported the frequency of anogenital findings (which included redness and swelling) decreased from 89% at less than 24 hours to 46% at greater than 72 hours after the assault. This is a particular concern among younger victims who may not report their assault in a timely fashion (Jones, Rossman, Wynn, et al., 2003).

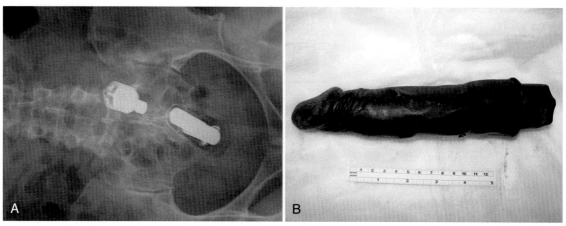

Figure 6-34
A, Radiograph of foreign object in large intestine after rectal sexual assault. B, Foreign object removed from large intestine during surgery.

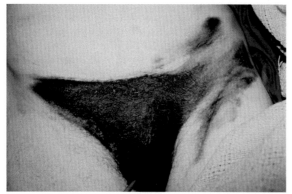

Figure 6-35
Extensive bruising over mons pubis after foreign object penetration.

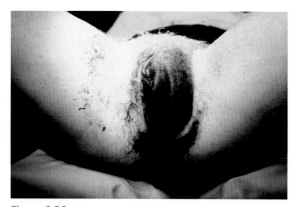

Figure 6-36
Large hematoma (13 cm x 14 cm x 10 cm) in left labia major and minor with bruising and abrasions after foreign object penetration.

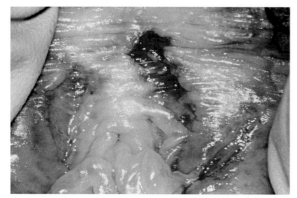

Figure 6-37
Multiple deep lacerations on labia minora after penetration with closed hand (i.e., fist).

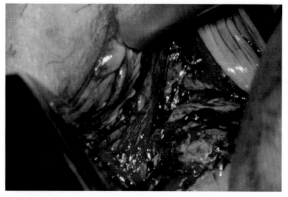

Figure 6-38
Extensive laceration of posterior and right lateral vaginal walls requiring surgical repair after penetration with closed hand (i.e., fist).

DELAYED MEDICAL FORENSIC EXAMINATION

Studies have suggested timing of the examination is the most significant predictor of abnormal anogenital findings in both children and adult victims of sexual assault (Adams, Knudson, 1996; Sachs, Chu, 2002). A 72- to 96-hour post-assault window is usually suggested as ideal for evidence collection and an initial police interview. However, Adams and colleagues (2001) determined the mean number of injury sites recorded did not vary according to the time interval between the assault and the examination. This suggests that time may enhance the visibility of some lesions, or that the severity of injury may cause victims to delay reporting. For example, anogenital contusions may not become visible for at least 48 hours.

In 2009, Olson, Burger, Dykstra, and colleagues compared the frequency and types of anogenital trauma in female victims examined acutely (less than 24 hours) with those who presented for forensic examination 24 to 120 hours following the sexual assault (Figure 6-39). A total of 2,799 cases presented to a community-based Nurse Examiner Program (NEP) during a 10-year study period. Twenty-eight percent of adult women and 33% of adolescent victims presented more than 24 hours after their assault. Victims who delayed seeking medical examination were younger, more likely to be assaulted by a known acquaintance or family member, and were less likely to report the assault to police. The frequency of anogenital lacerations and abrasions decreased from 71% at less than 24 hours to 28% at greater than 96 hours after the assault. Across all time periods adolescents had a consistently higher frequency of genital injuries compared with adults, but in both populations documented anogenital injuries steadily decreased each day after the assault by approximately 8%. At the 72-hour mark, 50% of adolescents and 38% of adult victims still had documented anogenital injuries.

ORAL PENETRATION

Oral injury may result from forced oral penile penetration or from external pressure such as grabbing and slapping. This may result in trauma to several structures within the mouth and lips.

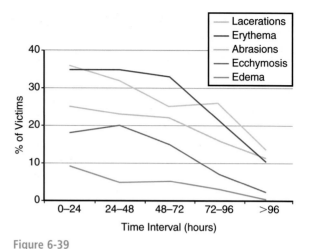

Figure 6-39

The types of documented anogenital injuries as a function of the time interval between the assault and the forensic examination. Over a 5-day period, genital abrasions and lacerations decreased by approximately 50%. Ecchymosis was actually more common at 48 hours and the degree of localized erythema did not significantly decrease until 72 hours post assault. (From Olson, M., Burger, C., Dykstra, D., et al. (2009). What happens at the 72-hour mark? Physical findings in sexual assault cases when victims delay reporting. *Annals of Emergency Medicine, 54*(3), S93. Used with permission of the authors.)

These include the external and inner lips, **frenulum** of the lips and tongue, **soft and hard palates**, tongue, **uvula**, teeth, and **buccal mucosa**. Types of injuries may include erythema, lacerations, contusions, **petechiae** (Figures 6-40 to 6-43), and loosened or avulsed teeth. Little research exists on physical findings associated with forced oral penetration. Damm and colleagues (1981) suggested a paucity of physical findings after forced oral contact. Soft palate injuries may be a direct result of negative pressure associated with oral penetration (Olshaker, Jackson, Smock, 2007) or from direct impact of the penis against the nasopharynx structures.

A detailed history will guide the examination of the **oral cavity**. The examination will require careful inspection of all the oral anatomical sites. Use of magnification may be helpful in detection of injuries. In sexual assaults with a history of oral penetration within 24 hours of the examination, it is recommended that oral cavity swabs be collected (Olshaker, Jackson, Smock, 2007). Sexual assault with oral penetration may result in exposure to sexually transmitted infections (STI). Prophylactic treatment of STI

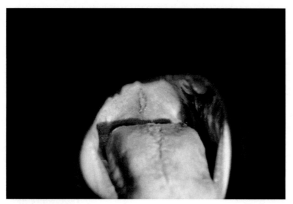

Figure 6-40
Soft palate abrasion with bruising.

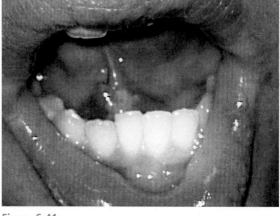

Figure 6-41
Frenulum laceration.

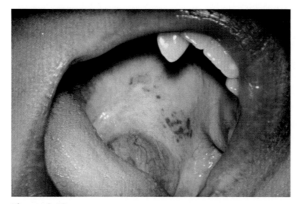

Figure 6-42
Soft palate bruising.

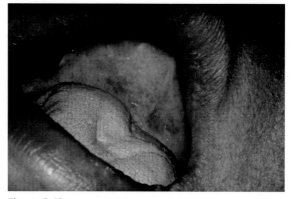

Figure 6-43
Soft palate bruising.

exposure should be considered and discussed with the patient. In summary, although oral trauma in the context of sexual assault is an area of needed research, the potential for trauma exists, and the oral cavity should be fully examined during the medical-forensic examination.

Interpretation and opinions regarding anogenital and oral injuries from sexual assault should be based on current scientific knowledge. It is imperative for forensic examiners to be familiar with the research surrounding anogenital and oral injury in reported sexual assaults, as well as in consensual sex. As the science evolves, so must the forensic examiner's **evidence-based practice**.

Key Terms

Adolescent
Anal canal
Anogenital
Anus
Bruise
Buccal mucosa
Cervix
Clitoral hood
Colposcope
Consensual sex
Digital penetration
Erythema
Evidence-based practice
Fellatio

References

Adams, J. A., Girardin, B., & Faugna, D. (2001). Adolescent sexual assault: Documentation of acute injuries using photo-colposcopy. *Journal of Adolescent and Pediatric Gynecology, 14*(4), 175–180.

Adams, J. A., & Knudson, S. (1996). Genital findings in adolescent girls referred for suspected sexual abuse. *Archives of Pediatrics and Adolescent Medicine, 150*(8), 850–857.

Alempijevic, D., Savic, S., Plavekic, S., & Jecmenica, D. (2006). Severity of injuries among sexual assault victims. *Journal of Forensic and Legal Medicine, 14*(5), 266–269.

Anderson, S., McClain, N., & Riviello, R. (2006). Genital findings of women after consensual and nonsensual intercourse. *Journal of Forensic Nursing, 2*(2), 59–65.

Baker, R. B., & Sommers, M. S. (2008). Relationship of genital injuries and age in adolescent and young adult rape survivors. *Journal of Obstetric, Gynecologic and Neonatal Nursing, 37*(3), 282–289.

Biggs, M., Stermac, L. E., & Divinsky, M. (1998). Genital injuries following sexual assault of women with and without prior sexual intercourse experience. *Canadian Medical Association Journal, 159*(1), 33–37.

Burgess, A. W., Hanrahan, N. P., & Baker, T. (2005). Forensic markers in elder female sexual abuse cases. *Clinics in Geriatric Medicine, 21*(2), 399–412.

Carey, R., Healy, C., & Elder, D. (2010). Foreign body sexual assault complicated by rectovaginal fistula. *Journal of Forensic and Legal Medicine, 17*(3), 161–163.

Cartwright, P. S. (1987). Factors that correlate with injury sustained by survivors of sexual assault. *Obstetrics and Gynecology, 70*(1), 44–46.

Chadwick, D. L., Berkowitz, C. D., Kerns, D., et al. (1989). *Color Atlas of Child Sexual Abuse*. Chicago: Year Book Medical Publishers.

Clay-Warner, J. (2002). Avoiding rape: The effects of protective actions and situational factors on rape outcome. *Violence and Victims, 17*(6), 691–705.

Coker, A. L., Walls, L. G., & Johnson, J. E. (1998). Risk factors for traumatic physical injury during sexual assaults for male and female victims. *Journal of Interpersonal Violence, 13*(5), 605–620.

Damm, D., White, D. & Brinker, M. (1981). Variations of palatal erythema secondary to fellatio. *Oral Surgery, 52*, 417.

Delacroix, J., Brown, J., Kadenhe-Chiweshe, et al. (2011). Rectal perforation secondary to rape and fisting in a female adolescent. *Pediatric Emergency Care, 27*(2), 116–119.

Del Bove, G., Stermac, L., & Bainbridge, D. (2005). Comparisons of sexual assault among older and younger women. *Journal of Elder Abuse and Neglect, 17*(3), 1–18.

Fain, D., & McCormick, G. (1989). Vaginal fisting as a cause of death. *The American Journal of Forensic Medicine and Pathology, 10*(1), 73–75.

Feldhaus, K. M., Houry, D., & Kaminsky, R. (2000). Lifetime sexual assault prevalence rates and reporting practices in an emergency department population. *Annals of Emergency Medicine, 36*(1), 23–27.

Gaffney, D. (2003). Genital injury and sexual assault. In A. P. Giardino, E. M. Datner, & J. B. Asher (Eds), *Sexual Assault. Victimization Across the Life Span: A Clinical Guide* (pp. 223–239). St Louis, MO: GW Medical Publishing.

Geist, R. (1988). Sexually related trauma. *Emergency Medicine Clinics of North America, 6*(3), 439–466.

Grossin, C., Sibille, I., Lorin de la Gradmaison, G., et al. (2003). Analysis of 418 cases of sexual assault. *Forensic Science International, 131*(2), 125–130.

Henry, T. (2010). Characteristics of sex-related homicides in Alaska. *Journal of Forensic Nursing, 6*(2), 57–65.

Jones, J. S., Genco, M., Dunnuck C, et al. (2003). Foley catheter balloon technique for visualizing the hymen in adolescent sexual assault victims. *Academic Emergency Medicine, 10*(9), 1001–1004.

Jones, J. S., Rossman, L., Diegel, R., et al. (2009). Sexual assault in postmenopausal women: Epidemiology and patterns of genital injury. *The American Journal of Emergency Medicine, 27*(8), 922–929.

Jones, J. S., Rossman, L., Hartman, M., & Alexander, C. (2004). Anogenital injuries in adolescents after consensual sexual intercourse. *Academy of Emergency Medicine, 10*(12), 1378–1383.

Jones, J. S., Rossman, L., Wynn, B., et al. (2003). Comparative analysis of adult versus adolescent sexual assault: Epidemiology and patterns of anogenital injury. *Academic Emergency Medicine, 10*(8), 872–877.

Lacey, H. B., & Roberts, R. (1991). Sexual assault on men. *International Journal of STD & AIDS, 2*(4), 258–260.

Lauber, A. A., & Souma, M. L. (1982). Use of toluidine blue dye for documentation of traumatic intercourse. *Obstetetrics & Gynecology, 60*(5), 644–648.

Lenahan, L., Ernst, A. & Johnson, B. (1998). Colposcopy in evaluation of the adult sexual assault victim. *American Journal of Emergency Medicine, 16*, 183–184.

Masho, S. W., & Alvanzo, A. (2009). Help-seeking behaviors of male sexual assault survivors. *American Journal of Men's Health, 20*(10), 1–6.

Massey, J., Garcia, C., & Emich, J. (1971). Management of sexually assaulted females. *Obstetrics & Gynecology, 38*(1), 29–36.

McCauley, J., Guzinski, G., Welch, R., et al. (1987). Toluidine blue dye in the corroboration of rape in the adult victim. *American Journal of Emergency Medicine, 5*(2), 105–108.

Olshaker, J., Jackson, C. & Smock, W. (2007). *Forensic Emergency Medicine* (p. 98). Philadelphia: Lippincott, Williams & Wilkins.

Olson, M., Burger, C., Dykstra, D., et al. (2009). What happens at the 72-hour mark? Physical findings in sexual assault cases when victims delay reporting. *Annals of Emergency Medicine, 54*(3), S93.

Orr, C., Clark, M., Hawley, D. et al. (1995). Fatal anorectal injuries: A series of four cases. *Journal of Forensic Sciences, 40*(2), 219–221.

Persaud, D. J., Squires, J. E., & Rubin-Remer, D. (1997). Use of Foley catheter to examine estrogenized hymens for evidence of sexual abuse. *Journal of Pediatric and Adolescent Gynecology, 10*(9), 83–85.

Poirier, M. P. (2002).Care of the female adolescent rape victim. *Pediatric Emergency Care, 18*(1), 53–58.

Rogers, A., McIntyre, S. L., Rossman, L., & Jones, J. S. (2008). The forensic rape examination: Is colposcopy really necessary? *Annals of Emergency Medicine, 52*(3), S63.

Rosay, A., & Henry, T. (2008). *A sexual assault nurse examiner study.* US Department of Justice document #224520. Retrieved from http://www.ncjrs.gov/pdffiles1/nij/grants/224520.pdf

Rossman, L., Jones, J. S., Dunnuck, C., et al. (2004). Genital trauma associated with forced digital penetration. *American Journal of Emergency Medicine, 22*(2), 101–104.

Rossman, L., Jones, J. S., Nelson-Horan, C. L., et al. (2000). Colposcopic genital findings in female sexual assault victims: Relationship to prior sexual intercourse experience. *Annals of Emergency Medicine, 36*(3), S83.

Sachs, C. J., & Chu, L. D. (2002). Predictors of genitorectal injury in female victims of suspected sexual assault. *Academic Emergency Medicine, 9*(2), 146–151.

Saltzman, L. E., Basile, K. C., Mahendra, R. R., et al. (2007). National estimates of sexual violence treated in emergency departments. *Annals of Emergency Medicine, 49*(2), 210–217.

Schwab, C. W., & Kauder, D. R. (1992). Trauma in the geriatric patient. *Archives of Surgery, 127*(6), 701–706.

Sedgwick, J. L. (2006). *Criminal victimization in the United States, 2005: statistical tables.* Washington DC: BJS Bulletin, NCJ 215244, Retrieved from http://bjs.ojp.usdoj.gov/content/pub/pdf/cvus05.pdf

Slaughter, L., & Brown, C. R. V. (1992). Colposcopy to establish physical findings in rape victims. *American Journal of Obstetrics and Gynecology, 166*(1), 83–86.

Slaughter, L., Brown, C. R. V., Crowley, S., & Peck, R. (1997). Patterns of genital injury in female sexual assault victims. *American Journal of Obstetrics and Gynecology, 176*(3), 609–616.

Snyder, H. (2000). *Sexual assault of young children as reported to law enforcement: Victim, incident, and offender characteristics.* BJS Bulletin, NCJ 182990, July 2000. Available at: http//www.ojp.usdoj.gov/bjs/pub/pdf/saycrle.pdf

Sommers, M. (2007). Defining patterns of genital injury from sexual assault: A review. *Trauma, Violence, & Abuse, 8*(3), 270–280.

Sommers, M., Schafer, J., Zink, T., et al. (2001). Injury patterns in women resulting from sexual assault. *Trauma, Violence, & Abuse, 2*(3), 240–258.

Sommers, M. S., Zink, T., Baker, R. B., et al. (2006). Effects of age and ethnicity on physical injury from rape. *Journal of Obstetrics, Gynecology, and Neonatal Nursing, 35*(2), 199–207.

Starling, S., & Jenny, C. (1997). Forensic examination of adolescent female genitalia: The Foley catheter technique. *Archives of Pediatric and Adolescent Medicine, 151*, 102–103.

Stermac, L., Del Bove, G., & Addison, M. (2004). Stranger and acquaintance sexual assault of adult males. *Journal of Interpersonal Violence, 19*(8), 901–915.

Stevens, J., Jones, J. S., Rossman, L., & Wynn, B. (2007). Effect of menstrual bleeding on the detection of anogenital injuries in sexual assault victims. *Annals of Emergency Medicine, 50*(1), S134.

Sturgiss, E., Tyson, A., & Parekh, V. (2010). Characteristics of sexual assaults in which adult victims report penetration by a foreign object. *Journal of Forensic and Legal Medicine, 17*(3), 140–142.

Sugar, N., Fine, D., & Eckert, L. (2004). Physical injury after sexual assault: Findings of a large case series. *American Journal of Obstetrics and Gynecology, 190*(1), 71–76.

U.S. Department of Justice, Office on Violence Against Women. (2004*). A national protocol for sexual assault medical forensic examinations (adults/adolescents)*. Retrieved from http//www.ncjrs.org/pdffiles1/ovw/206554.pdf

Walker, J., Archer, J., & Davies, M. (2005). Effects of rape on men: A descriptive analysis. *Archives of Sexual Behavior, 34*(1), 69–80.

CHAPTER 7

POSTMORTEM SEXUAL ASSAULT EXAMINATIONS

Tara Henry

Sexual assault combined with homicide represents one of the most extreme forms of violence perpetrated against women. A variety of terms are used to refer to this form of violence including sexual homicide, sexual assault homicide, rape homicide, or sex-related homicide. For the purpose of this chapter, **sex-related homicide** will be used. There is a paucity of data in the United States for this type of crime; therefore, it is unknown how often sex-related homicides occur. It is estimated that sex-related homicides account for 1% to 4% of homicides in North America (Roberts, Grossman, 1993; Meloy, 2000). According to Henry (2010), it is likely that many sex-related homicides are not identified, resulting in significantly underestimated prevalence data.

A sex-related homicide should be considered when there is an indication of sexual activity at the crime scene or on the body of the victim (Geberth, 2010). Indicators that should cue forensic examiners to suspect a sex-related homicide are numerous. The body may be positioned in a sexual manner; clothing may be missing or arranged to expose the breasts, buttocks or genitalia; seminal fluid may be present; foreign objects used for penetration may be left behind; and injury or mutilation of the genitalia, anus, buttocks or breasts may be visible (Henry, 2010; Geberth, 2010; Ressler, Burgess, Douglas, 1992).

COLLABORATION

For living victims of sexual assault, healthcare providers recognize best practice is to provide access to a **medical-forensic examination** by a forensic examiner specialized in caring for patients affected by sexual violence. The **forensic examiner** may be a registered nurse, advanced nurse practitioner, physician, or physician assistant. Forensic nurses have taken a leadership role in healthcare's response to sexual violence, and many communities have established **Sexual Assault Nurse Examiner (SANE)** programs to provide specialized forensic nursing care to patients who report a sexual assault. National and international guidelines have been established to provide evidence-based standards of practice for healthcare practitioners who perform sexual assault medical-forensic examinations

on living victims (U.S. Department of Justice, 2004; World Health Organization, 2003). The use of various tools to enhance visualization and documentation of genital injuries, such as a **colposcope** and/or digital camera with macro lens, and toluidine blue dye, are routinely used during medical-forensic examinations of living sexual assault victims. Few advancements have been made to utilize similar specialists and technology for deceased sexual assault victims (Slaughter, 2006); however, this is beginning to change as more communities recognize the value of **forensic pathologists** partnering with sexual assault specialists to respond to sex-related homicide cases (Henry, 2010; Willoughby, Heger, Rogers, Sathyavagiswaran, 2010; Crowley, 2011).

As collaboration occurs among forensic pathologists and forensic nurses or other sexual assault specialists, it is important that roles are defined and protocols are established for the postmortem sexual assault examination.

Some communities have a forensic nurse respond to the crime scene to assist with evidence collection and examination of the body at the scene (Diegel, 2011). Other communities contract with a forensic nurse to assist with evidence collection and examination of the body at autopsy (Henry, 2010), and some communities have forensic nurses employed as coroners or as death investigators with the local medical examiner's office (Lynch, 2011).

EVIDENCE COLLECTION

"**Physical evidence** encompasses any and all objects that can establish that a crime has been committed or can provide a link between a crime and its victim or a crime and its perpetrator (Saferstein, 2007, p. 33)."

Sexual assault evidence collection kits, which are usually available through local or state crime laboratories, assist with the collection and packaging of **forensic samples**. The kits are composed of a series of envelopes, paper bindles, swabs, microscope slides, and clothing bags. Some kits also contain fingernail scrapers, combs, and urine and blood specimen containers. If a sexual assault evidence collection kit is not available, the forensic examiner will need to gather the items necessary for collecting and packaging forensic samples per agency protocol. Samples collected by the forensic examiner while at the crime scene will require additional equipment and supplies to facilitate identification and collection of evidence from the body.

> Routine samples should be collected in a sex-related homicide regardless of the examination location (crime scene or medical examiner's office). According to Henry (2010), samples that should be obtained during a postmortem sexual assault examination include clothing, tape lifts, miscellaneous hairs, fibers, debris, pulled scalp hair, pulled pubic hair, swabs of the neck, breasts, mouth, external genitalia, vagina, cervix, anus, and rectum. Swabs should also be obtained of blood spatter, any areas of fluorescence seen with an alternative light source, and areas of bruising that might yield skin cell transfer from the suspect.

NON-GENITAL INJURY

> Sex-related homicides often have significant **non-genital injury** demonstrating the extreme level of violence that occurred.

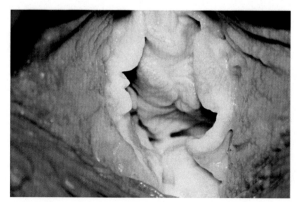

Figure 7-1
Normal postmortem hymen and medial aspect labia minora.

The most frequent **cause of death** is **strangulation**, followed by **blunt force trauma, stabbing** and **gunshot wounds** (Abrahams, Martin, Jewkes, et al., 2008; Roberts, Grossman, 1993; Van Patten, Delhauer, 2007). According to Spitz (1993), when strangulation is present, a sexual motive to the crime must be considered, especially if the victim is female, regardless of the age. **Bite marks** are also associated with sex-related homicide (Abrahams, Martin, Jewkes, et al., 2008).

> The head, neck, and chest are the most common non-genital sites of injury, likely a result of the intense fury felt by the assailant combined with such intimate physical contact with the victim.

Although non-genital injury is often present in sex-related homicides, minimal or absent non-genital injury does not rule out the possibility of a sex-related homicide. Henry (2010) found **anogenital** injury alone was significant enough to cause death in 22% of sex-related homicide victims.

ANOGENITAL EXAMINATION

Performing an **anogenital examination** postmortem is not significantly different than an anogenital examination of a living patient.

> If the anogenital tissue has minimal to no decomposition present, the examiner can manipulate the tissue without difficulty.

In the absence of circulating blood, the tissue is pale (Figure 7-1) and cool to the touch. If the body was exposed to a freezing environment, such as left outdoors in freezing temperatures or placed in a freezer, the tissue feels similar to dough once the body has thawed.

> It is not unusual for the anogenital orifices to gape open, and care should be taken not to misinterpret this normal finding as evidence of sexual assault (Figure 7-2).

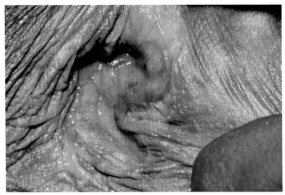

Figure 7-2
Normal postmortem anal dilation; anal canal visible with feces leaking.

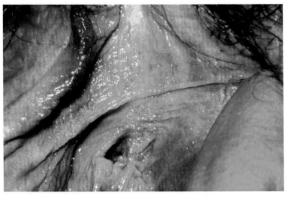

Figure 7-3
Normal postmortem urethral gaping; urine may leak with minimal tissue manipulation.

A gaping **urethra** (Figure 7-3) will often leak urine from a full bladder once manipulation of the genital tissue begins. With the body in a supine position for the anogenital examination, a steady stream of urine may leak into the vagina or anal canal, interrupt external genital trace evidence collection, or cause some difficulty obtaining colposcopic photographs. Loose stool, if present in the rectum, may also leak from a dilated anus. When there is minimal or no feces present, the **anal canal** and rectum can be visualized through the dilated anus (Figure 7-4). An anus that is closed prior to **anoscope** examination often remains open after the anoscope is removed, as will the anal canal (Figure 7-5).

To prevent misinterpretation of postmortem anogenital findings, it is critical for the sexual assault specialist to obtain initial and ongoing education in normal postmortem tissue changes, postmortem artifacts, as well as postmortem identification and interpretation of wounds.

There are many textbooks, articles, and training available to acquire this general knowledge; however, minimal information is available regarding "normal" postmortem anogenital appearance, particularly when visualized with a colposcope (Henry, 2010; Crowley,

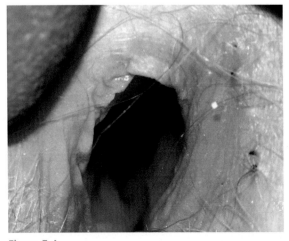

Figure 7-4
Normal postmortem anal dilation; anal canal and rectum visible.

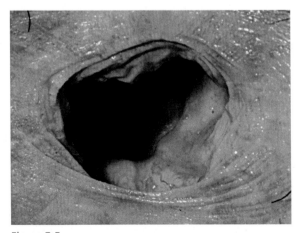

Figure 7-5
Postmortem anal and rectal dilation after anoscope removal; normal finding.

2011). Some workshops and lectures have been available at forensic science and forensic nursing scientific assemblies to educate colleagues on this subject; however, it will be essential to have more education opportunities, resources, and research available to sexual assault specialists who expand their clinical practice to include postmortem sexual assault examinations.

RIGOR MORTIS

Rigor mortis, also known as **rigidity**, is a temporary stiffening of the muscles after death. It is noticeable in the smaller muscle groups first, usually within 2 to 4 hours after death, and observable in the larger muscle groups 6 to 12 hours after death. Rigor mortis is caused by the loss of **adenosine triphosphate (ATP)** regeneration and an increase in lactic acid in the muscles after death.

This results in a locking of the muscle proteins, **actin** and **myosin**, which produces muscle stiffening (Knight, 1996; Spitz, 1993). When rigor is present, the **labia majora** may feel less supple with manipulation, the cervix is less mobile, and the vaginal walls can be less pliable. Occasionally this makes it difficult to open and position a speculum for visualization of the cervix (Figures 7-6 and 7-7) and vaginal walls. Although rigor affects the elasticity of the vaginal walls, it does not affect the appearance (Figures 7-8 and 7-9).

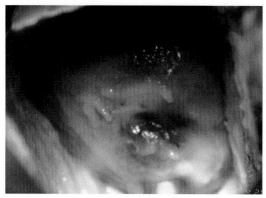

Figure 7-7
Normal postmortem cervix; speculum partially open due to rigor.

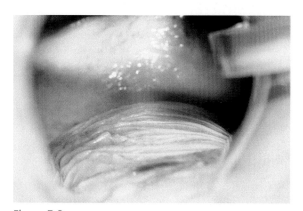

Figure 7-8
Normal postmortem posterior vaginal wall.

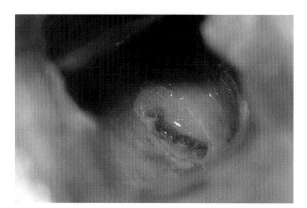

Figure 7-6
Normal postmortem cervix; speculum partially open due to rigor.

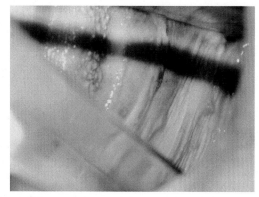

Figure 7-9
Normal postmortem right lateral vaginal wall; rugae visible.

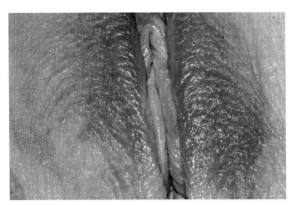

Figure 7-10
Labia majora with lividity; normal finding.

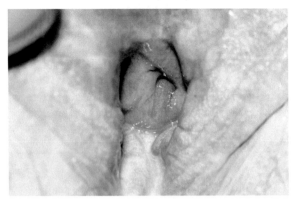

Figure 7-11
Periurethra with generalized lividity; normal finding.

LIVOR MORTIS

Livor mortis, also known as **lividity** or postmortem hypostasis can be noticeable within 30 minutes after death, but may take longer. It generally reaches maximum coloration 8 to 12 hours after death, at which time it is considered "fixed" (DiMaio, DiMaio, 1993). Lividity is caused from the settling of blood via gravity after circulation ceases.

Lividity ranges from pink to bright red in color, but can be bluish-purple.

Clinicians unfamiliar with the appearance of lividity on the anogenitalia may misinterpret this normal finding as bruising.

Forensic nurses and other sexual assault specialists performing postmortem sexual assault examinations must be familiar with the various manifestations of anogenital lividity (Figures 7-10 to 7-15) and collaborate with the forensic pathologist to differentiate lividity from bruising. A bruise will not blanch when pressure is applied to the tissue. An incision into the questionable area can help confirm bruising. An incised bruise shows diffuse hemorrhage into the soft

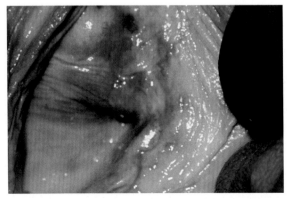

Figure 7-12
Lividity visible on left labia minor, hymen, and anterior vaginal wall from the 1 o'clock to the 4 o'clock positions.

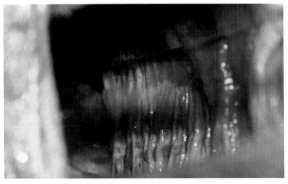

Figure 7-13
Lividity on left lateral vaginal wall visualized with speculum in place; normal finding.

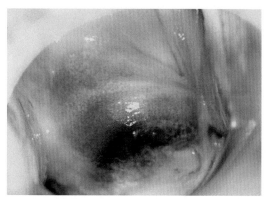

Figure 7-14
Lividity on anterior portion of cervix visualized with speculum in place; normal finding.

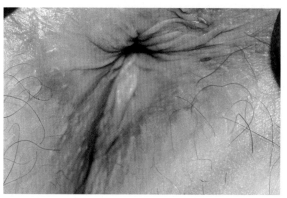

Figure 7-15
Lividity on anus from the 3 o'clock to the 9 o'clock positions; normal finding.

tissue, whereas incised lividity shows blood confined to the vessels without hemorrhage into the soft tissue (Figure 7-16) (DiMaio, DiMaio, 1993).

DECOMPOSITION

Decomposition is the disintegration of body tissues after death as a result of the autolysis of cells and putrefaction.

Putrefaction occurs when the bacterial flora of the gastrointestinal tract invade the vascular system and spread throughout the body. Putrefaction is first noticeable as a greenish discoloration of the lower quadrants of the abdomen then spreads throughout the body, most often next affecting the head, neck, and chest. **Bloating** then occurs from bacterial gas formation, followed by vesicle development (Figure 7-17) and skin and hair slippage (Figure 7-18) (DiMaio, DiMaio, 1993; Knight, 1996).

Colposcopic anogenital examination can be performed even with decomposition present; however, the examiner must not confuse **skin slippage** with abrasions (Figures 7-19 to 7-21).

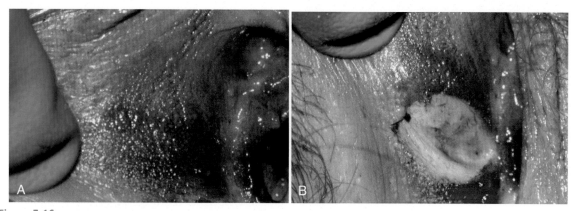

Figure 7-16
A, Right labium minus, medial aspect with dark red discoloration at the 9 o'clock position. B, Right labium minus, medial aspect with dark red discoloration at the 9 o'clock position incised; no hemorrhage in tissue confirms lividity; normal finding.

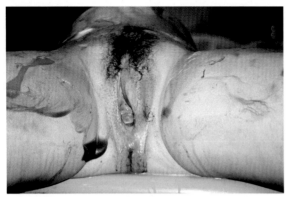

Figure 7-17
Putrefaction. Note green discoloration on labia majora and perineum, bloating of left labium majus, vesicular formation on thighs and groin.

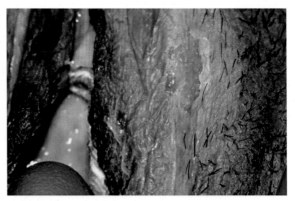

Figure 7-19
Left labium majus with skin slippage from the 2 o'clock to 3 o'clock positions; normal postmortem change.

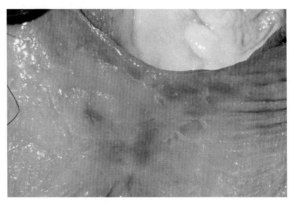

Figure 7-20
Posterior fourchette and perineum with skin slippage; normal postmortem change.

The sexual assault specialist should be prepared to observe several postmortem changes to the ano-genitalia (Figure 7-22) and recognize these as normal findings.

MUMMIFICATION AND ADIPOCERE

Mummification of the body can occur in environments with low humidity and good ventilation. Although this postmortem change typically occurs over the entire body, drying of certain parts of the body such as the conjunctiva, fingers and toes, scrotum, labia majora, and **labia minora** often occur without mummification of the body. Drying of these tissues causes a brownish discoloration and parchment-like appearance (Figure 7-23) and can be mistaken for bruising (Spitz, 1993).

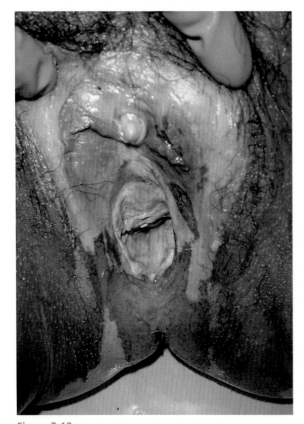

Figure 7-18
Putrefaction; hair and skin slippage of entire external genitalia, anus, buttocks.

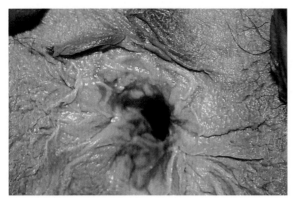

Figure 7-21
Anus with skin slippage; dilated, anal canal visible; normal post-mortem change.

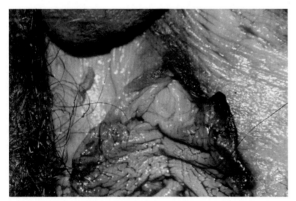

Figure 7-23
Clitoral hood with drying from the 12 o'clock to 2 o'clock positions. Note the dark, parchment-like appearance.

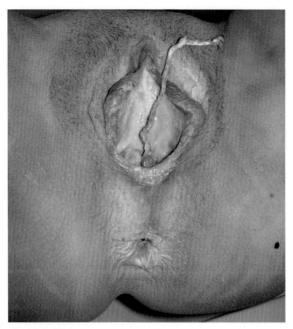

Figure 7-22
Postmortem anogenitalia with lividity, green-black discoloration, skin slippage; tampon string visible.

Adipocere is a wax-like substance formed by the hydrolysis and hydrogenation of body fat. It develops in environments with high humidity and is often seen on bodies that have been in wet graves (Knight, 1996; Spitz, 1993). If adipocere is formed on the anogenitalia (Figure 7-24), a postmortem anogenital examination by the sexual assault expert is unlikely to be beneficial.

INSECTS

Flies are the most common type of insect associated with decomposing bodies (DiMaio, DiMaio, 1993).

Maggots, the larval stage of flies, are quite destructive to the body, particularly to wounds.

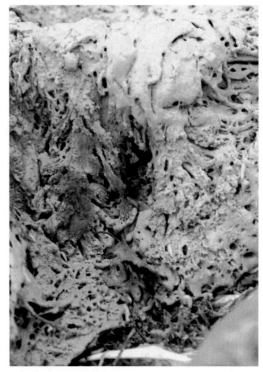

Figure 7-24
Adipocere of the anogenitalia.

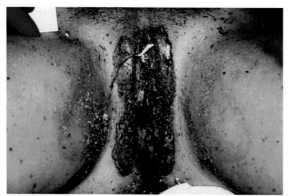

Figure 7-25
External genitalia with maggots. Note the burrowing and tunnels on labia majora and perineum.

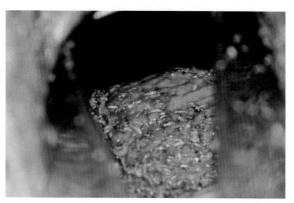

Figure 7-26
Large concentration of maggots in vagina; no injury was present after removal of maggots.

Maggots primarily concentrate on the natural openings of the body, such as the eyes, nostrils, mouth, genitalia and anus, and in open wounds. They burrow beneath the skin creating tunnels (Figure 7-25), which admit air and access to other external microorganisms and accelerate the decomposition process (Knight, 1996). When a large amount of maggots are concentrated in a specific area, it is likely that a wound preexisted in that location (Spitz, 1993).

> Since the anogenital area is a normal location to observe significant concentrations of maggots, caution should be used when interpreting the presence of maggots at this site because it does not necessarily mean injuries are, or were, present (Figure 7-26).

After initial photographs have been taken and forensic samples obtained, the maggots should be gently wiped or washed off the anogenitalia so any areas of concern can be more thoroughly assessed.

COLPOSCOPE

The use of a colposcope as a tool to enhance visualization of anogenital injury during medical-forensic examination of living sexual assault victims is well established. There is an abundance of literature that discusses the presence and absence of anogenital injury from reported sexual assaults. In 1997, Slaughter and colleagues published seminal research on anogenital injuries seen with a colposcope during sexual assault examinations (Slaughter, Brown, Crowley, 1997). Since that time numerous studies have been published describing the types, sites, and patterns of anogenital injury identified with colposcopic examination of living sexual assault victims. Traditionally, direct visualization and histological sampling of injury have been the primary postmortem anogenital examination methods used for sex-related homicides. Bays and Lewman (1992) have used a colposcope and toluidine blue dye in postmortem child sexual abuse examinations. In more recent years, Crowley (2004) and Elder (2007) have suggested the use of a colposcope or other magnification to enhance injury detection and photodocumentation in postmortem sexual assault examinations.

TOLUIDINE BLUE DYE

Toluidine blue dye, a nuclear stain, is frequently used to highlight lacerations and abrasions at certain anatomical sites on the anogenitalia of living sexual assault victims. Positive results are indicated by the nucleated cells staining dark purple-blue, whereas negative results are indicated by no staining, or a diffuse light purple-blue stain. Postive toluidine blue dye uptake is not diagnostic of trauma. A positive result simply means there are exposed nucleated cells. Inflammation, mucous, cancer, and numerous other categories of benign disease that result in exposed nucleated cells can have a positive toluidine blue dye stain (Collins, Hansen, Theriot, 1966).

Currently, there are no published studies that investigate the effect of postmortem changes and artifacts on toluidine blue dye staining. Since the efficacy of toluidine blue dye staining in the postmortem setting is primarily anecdotal, interpretation of results should be made with caution.

Figures 7-27 to 7-29 show examples of toluidine blue dye application to anogenital injuries identified in postmortem sexual assault examinations performed within 36 hours of when the victim was last seen alive.

INJURY

The vast majority of literature available on anogenital injury observed in sex-related homicide cases describe the injury locations in general terms, such as external

genitalia, introitus, or vagina instead of the exact anatomical site. Sexual assault specialists should assess and document anogenital injury at the specific anogenital site similar to documentation in nonfatal sexual assault cases. These anatomical sites are mons pubis, labia majora, labia minora, clitoral hood, clitoris, periurethra, hymen, fossa navicularis, posterior fourchette, perineum, vaginal walls (anterior, posterior, lateral), cervix, anus, anal canal, and rectum.

To date, there is only one study published describing the types, sites, and patterns of anogenital injury seen with colposcopic examination of deceased sexual assault victims (Henry, 2010). In this study Henry reported anogenital injury in 58% of sex-related homicide cases. The most common sites of injury were the labia minora, (Figure 7-30) posterior fourchette (Figure 7-31), hymen (Figure 7-32), and anus (Figure 7-33). Lacerations were the most common type of

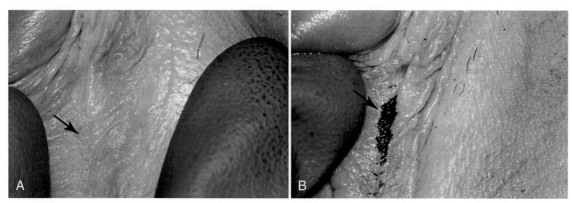

Figure 7-27
A, Laceration at left labium minus/majus junction. B, Same laceration as seen in Figure 7-27A with toluidine blue dye.

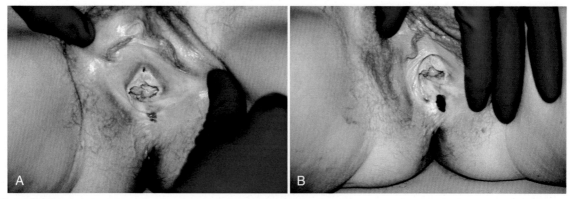

Figure 7-28
A, Laceration on perineum and posterior fourchette. B, Same laceration as seen in Figure 7-28A with toluidine blue dye.

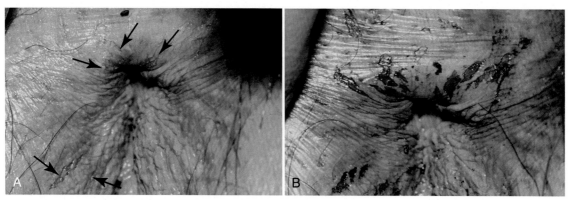

Figure 7-29
A, Multiple lacerations on perineum and anus. B, Same lacerations as seen in Figure 7-29A with toluidine blue dye.

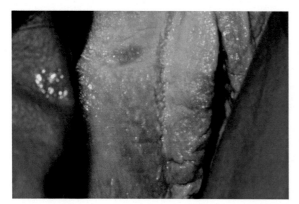

Figure 7-30
Laceration on right labium minus/majus junction.

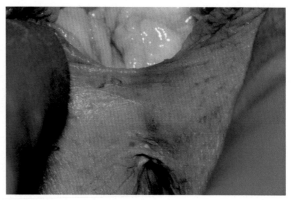

Figure 7-31
Laceration on posterior fourchette.

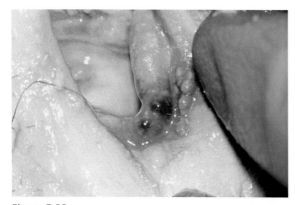

Figure 7-32
Bruising on hymen.

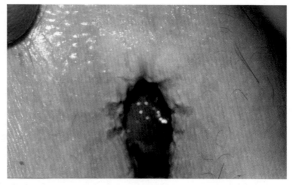

Figure 7-33
Multiple lacerations in stellate pattern on anus; anal dilation normal postmortem finding.

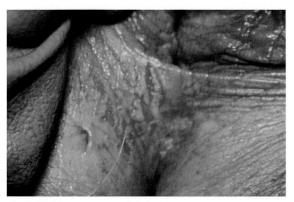

Figure 7-34
Multiple lacerations on perineum and posterior fourchette.

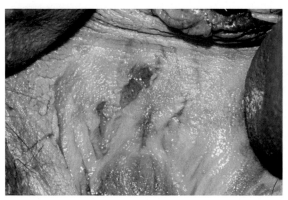

Figure 7-35
Multiple lacerations on labia minora above urethra. Underlying redness is lividity and should not be mistaken for bruising.

injury (Figures 7-34 to 7-36), followed by abrasions (Figures 7-37 and 7-38) then bruises (Figures 7-39 and 7-40). The lacerations occurred most often on the labia minora, anus, and posterior fourchette. Abrasions occurred most often on the labia minora, perineum, anus, and labia majora. Bruises occurred most often on the labia minora and hymen. It is not unusual to have multiple sites and types of anogenital injury in sex-related homicides (Figures 7-41 and 7-42).

Similar to nonfatal sexual assaults, anogenital injuries are generally of minor severity; however, Henry (2010) found in 22% of sex-related homicides, the anogenital injuries from blunt force trauma were significant enough to result in death (Figures 7-43 and 7-44).

Injuries of this gravity are usually associated with penetration with a foreign object. Severe injuries such as these should be closely inspected for rectal or peritoneal perforation (Figures 7-45 and 7-46). For extensive vaginal or rectal injuries, the anogenitalia should be removed en bloc and dissected to determine extent of injury (Figure 7-47).

Superficial anogenital abrasions and lacerations observed in living victims of sexual assault often have no bleeding or bruising associated with them. This is also the case in postmortem sexual assault anogenital findings. Occasionally this may make it difficult to determine antemortem versus postmortem injury occurrence.

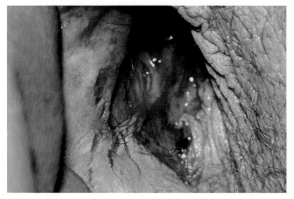

Figure 7-36
Lacerations extending through anal canal into rectum.

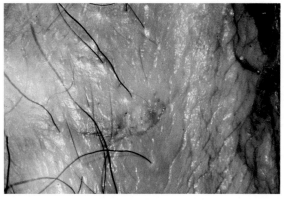

Figure 7-37
Abrasion on right labium majus.

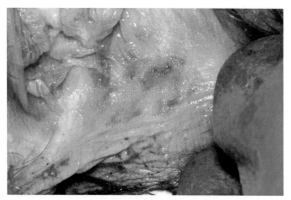

Figure 7-38
Abrasions on medial aspect left labium minus.

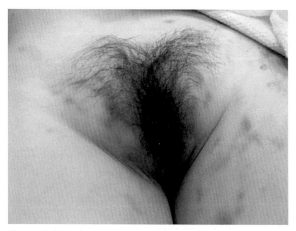

Figure 7-39
Bruising on mons pubis and inner thighs.

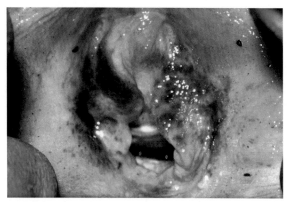

Figure 7-40
Bruising on hymen; debris on labia minora.

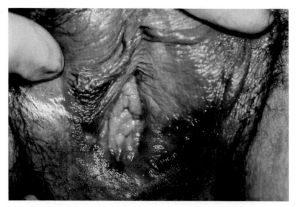

Figure 7-41
Bruising and lacerations on left labium minus, posterior fourchette, and fossa navicularis.

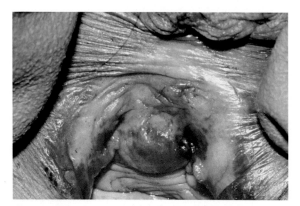

Figure 7-42
Lacerations and bruising on labia minora and periurethra.

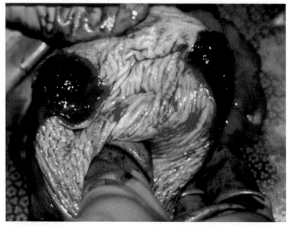

Figure 7-43
Lacerations on bilateral vaginal walls; victim deceased from exsanguination.

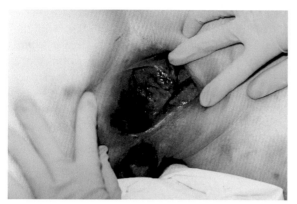

Figure 7-44
Laceration extends through anus, anal canal, rectum, and 4 inches into right buttock tissue; victim deceased from exsanguination.

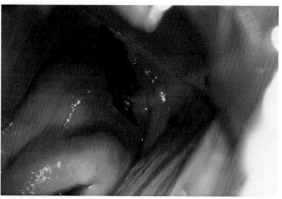

Figure 7-45
Laceration anterior and left lateral vaginal fornices; perforation into peritoneal cavity; debris present.

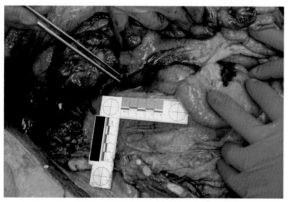

Figure 7-46
Piece of wood from broken tree branch in abdominal cavity; rectal perforation present.

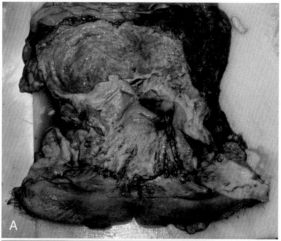

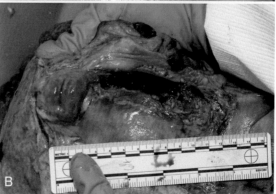

Figure 7-47
A, Anogenitalia en bloc and dissected to expose vaginal walls. Note sutured laceration on left lateral wall from medical intervention; multiple other lacerations on posterior and right lateral vaginal wall; bruising throughout. B, Anogenitalia en bloc and dissected to expose vaginal walls; sutures removed from left lateral wall laceration shown in Figure 7-47A. Note blood clot from torn artery.

In some jurisdictions this determination can make a difference in the criminal charges associated with the homicide (e.g., sexual assault is considered a felony, whereas misconduct with a corpse is considered a misdemeanor.) An abrasion or laceration that extends deeper into the dermis and facia should have some associated bleeding or bruising if sustained antemortem. The lack of this additional finding should cause the examiner to suspect the injury was sustained postmortem (Figures 7-48 to 7-50).

Microscopic examination of tissue samples by the forensic pathologist may be helpful when antemortem versus postmortem injury is questionable.

DOCUMENTATION

Most colposcopes have photographic capabilities.

Whether using a colposcope or handheld camera, photographs should be taken during the postmortem anogenital examination.

Photodocumentation should be taken of each anatomical site to document the presence or absence of injury, postmortem changes, or artifacts. Photographs should be obtained of any foreign material before removal for forensic evidence (Figure 7-51), before and after cleaning of tissue, before and after application of toluidine blue dye if used, and of all anogenital injury.

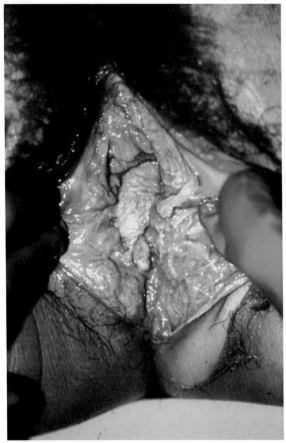

Figure 7-48
Laceration extending through perineum and posterior vaginal wall into anus and rectum. Note lack of hemorrhaging throughout; caused postmortem from penetration with shotgun barrel.

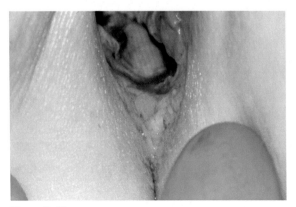

Figure 7-49
Laceration extending into perineum and posterior vaginal wall. Note lack of hemorrhaging throughout; caused from postmortem penetration.

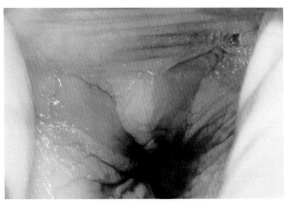

Figure 7-50
Laceration on anus extending into anal canal. Note lack of hemorrhaging throughout; caused from postmortem penetration with a bottle.

Written documentation should include the known history of circumstances surrounding the death, any known pertinent medical history, non-genital and anogenital examination findings, methods of examination used, and a list of clothing and other specimens collected for forensic evidence.

If supplemental documentation is needed, an addendum should be added to the original report.

The forensic nurse and other sexual assault specialists have a responsibility to maintain their professional practice standards and follow state licensure regulations for their discipline.

As protocols are developed for collaboration between the forensic pathologist and sexual assault clinician, these responsibilities should be understood.

There will be areas of overlap with documentation because both the sexual assault examiner and the forensic pathologist are professionally responsible for creating written medical-forensic records.

This is no different than collaborations and consultations between healthcare providers caring for living patients. Like any professional partnership, mutual respect for each person's discipline, good communication, established role boundaries and responsibilities, and a common goal help to create a strong foundation for successful collaboration.

FUTURE

Deceased victims should be afforded comprehensive sexual assault examinations that utilize the most current technology, standards, and expertise presently available to living victims of sexual assault.

As more communities establish collaborative relationships among forensic pathologists and forensic nurses, or other sexual assault specialists to provide this service, it is imperative that these clinicians also address the disparity in research surrounding postmortem sexual assault evaluations and help build an evidence-based foundation for clinical practice in medical-forensic examinations of sex-related homicide victims.

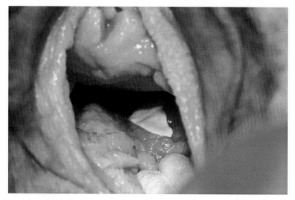

Figure 7-51
Condom piece on posterior vaginal wall matching missing piece of broken condom at crime scene.

Key Terms

Actin
Adenosine triphosphate
Adipocere
Anal canal
Anogenital
Anogenital examination
Anoscope
Anus
Bite mark
Bloating
Blunt force trauma
Cause of death
Cervix
Clitoral hood
Clitoris
Colposcope
Decomposition
External genitalia
Forensic examiner
Forensic pathologist
Forensic sample
Fossa navicularis
Gunshot wound

Hymen
Labia majora
Labia minora
Lividity
Livor mortis
Maggot
Medical-forensic examination
Mons pubis
Mummification
Myosin
Non-genital injury
Perineum
Periurethra
Physical evidence
Posterior fourchette
Putrefaction
Rectum
Rigidity
Rigor mortis
Sex-related homicide
Sexual Assault Nurse Examiner (SANE) program
Skin slippage
Stabbing
Strangulation
Toluidine blue dye
Urethra
Vagina

References

Abrahams, N., Martin, L., Jewkes, R., et al. (2008). The epidemiology and the pathology of suspected rape homicide in South Africa. *Forensic Science International, 178,* 132–138.

Bays, J., & Lewman, L. (1992). Toluidine blue in the detection at autopsy of perineal and anal lacerations in victims of sexual abuse. *Archives of Pathology and Laboratory Medicine, 116,* 620–621.

Collins, C., Hansen, L., & Theriot, E. (1966). A clinical stain for use in selecting biopsy sites in patients with vulvar disease. *Obstetrics and Gynecology, 28*(2), 158–163.

Crowley, S. (2004). A mobile system for postmortem genital examinations with colposcopy: SART-to-go. *Journal of Forensic Science, 49*(6), 1–9.

Crowley, S. (2011). Postmortem sexual assault evaluation. In V. Lynch, & J. Duval (Eds.), *Forensic Nursing Science* (2nd ed., pp. 234–248). St. Louis, MO: Elsevier Mosby.

Diegel, R. (2011). Medical evidence recovery at the death scene. In V. Lynch, & J. Duval (Eds.), *Forensic Nursing Science* (2nd ed., pp. 222–233). St. Louis, MO: Elsevier Mosby.

DiMaio, D., & DiMaio, V. (1993). *Forensic Pathology.* Boca Raton, FL: CRC Press.

Elder, D. (2007). Interpretation of anogenital findings in the living child: Implications for paediatric forensic autopsy. *Journal of Forensic and Legal Medicine, 14,* 482–488.

Geberth, V. (2010). *Sex-related homicide and death investigation.* Boca Raton, FL: CRC Press.

Henry, T. (2010). Characteristics of sex-related homicides in Alaska. *Journal of Forensic Nursing, 6*(2), 57–65.

Knight, B. (1996). *Forensic Pathology.* (2nd ed.). New York: Arnold.

Lynch, V. (2011). Forensic nurse examiners in death investigation. In V. Lynch, & J. Duval, *Forensic Nursing Science* (2nd ed., pp. 195–211). St. Louis, MO: Elsevier Mosby.

Meloy, J. (2000). The nature and dynamics of sexual homicide: An integrative review. *Aggression and Violent Behavior, 5*(1), 1–22.

Ressler, R., Burgess, A., & Douglas, J. (1992). *Sexual homicide patterns and motives.* New York: Free Press.

Roberts, J., & Grossman, M. (1993). Sexual homicide in Canada: A descriptive analysis. *Annals of Sex Research, 6,* 5–25.

Saferstein, R. (2007). *Criminalistics: An introduction to forensic science.* Upper Saddle River, NJ: Prentice Hall.

Slaughter, L. (2006). Binocular microscopy in sexual assault examination. In V. Lynch, *Forensic Nursing* (pp. 157–169). St. Louis, MO: Elsevier Mosby.

Slaughter, L., Brown, C., Crowley, S., & Peck, R. (1997). Patterns of genital injury in female sexual assault victims. *American Journal of Obstetrics and Gynecology, 176*(3), 609–615.

Spitz, W. (Ed.). (1993). *Medicolegal investigation of death: Guidelines for the application of pathology to crime investigation.* (3rd ed.). Springfield, IL: Charles C. Thomas.

U. S. Department of Justice. (2004). *A national protocol for sexual assault medical forensic examination: Adults/adolescents.* Washington, DC: Office on Violence Against Women.

Van Patten, I., & Delhauer, P. (2007). Sexual homicide: A spatial analysis of 25 years of deaths in Los Angeles. *Journal of Forensic Science, 52*(5), 1129–1141.

Willoughby, V., Heger, A., Rogers, C., & Sathyavagiswaran, L. (2010). Sexual assault documentation program. *American Journal of Forensic Medicine and Pathology, 31*(3), 1–4.

World Health Organization. (2003). *Guidelines for medicolegal care for victims of sexual violence.* Geneva: World Health Organization.

Abrasion: Wound caused by the scraping or rubbing away of skin.

Abscess: A pus-filled cavity surrounded by inflamed tissue.

Accessory glands: Glands that assist organs in accomplishing their function.

Actin: A protein found in muscle tissue that assists with contraction and relaxation.

Adenosine triphosphate: A chemical compound that transports energy within cells for metabolism.

Adipocere: A wax-like postmortem substance caused by fat decomposition.

Adipose tissue: A collection of fat cells.

Adolescent: A person in the process of adolescence.

Alternative light source: A term used to refer to a laser light source or ultraviolet light over 400 nm.

Anal canal: The terminal end of the large intestine located between the rectum and anus.

Angiokeratoma: Benign vascular lesion on the skin characterized by small marks of red to blue color.

Annular: Ring shaped.

Anogenital: Relates to the anus and genitalia region.

Anogenital examination: Examination of the anus and genitalia.

Anogenital injury: Wound on the anus or genitalia.

Anorectal: Relates to the anus and rectum.

Anoscope: A small, tubular speculum used to visualize the anal canal.

Anterior commissure: Anterior junction of the labia majora at the base of the symphysis pubis.

Anus: Opening at the terminal end of the anal canal.

Atrophic: Wasting away or decrease in size of tissue.

Avulsion: Wound caused by the pulling or tearing away of a part of the body.

Bacterial vaginosis: Infection of the vagina caused by an imbalance of naturally occurring bacterial flora.

Bartholin glands: Small mucous-secreting glands located in the posterior vestibule.

Bartholin gland cyst: A fluid-filled sac formed when the Bartholin gland is blocked.

Bilirubin: Yellowish pigment formed when heme is removed from hemoglobin during the breakdown of red blood cells.

Biliverdin: Greenish bile pigment formed by the breakdown of hemoglobin.

Bite mark: Patterned wound caused by the act of biting.

Bloating: Swelling or filling with gas.

Blunt force trauma: Wound caused by blunt force.

Bruise: A wound that occurs when blunt force ruptures or tears a blood vessel resulting in leakage of blood into the tissue. Also known as a contusion.

Buccal mucosa: Mucous membrane lining the inside of the cheek.

Bulbourethral glands: Glands in the urethral sphincter at the base of the penis that contribute a small amount of fluid to semen. Also known as Cowper glands.

Bulla: An elevated collection of clear, serous fluid greater than 1 cm in diameter.

Candidiasis: An infection caused by a species of *Candida*, usually *Candida* albicans.

Cause of death: Any injury or disease that results in a person dying.

Cervix: Neck or narrow, lower portion of the uterus.

Cherry angioma: Red, flat, benign vascular lesion less than 4 mm in diameter.

Chlamydia trachomatis: Gram-negative bacteria responsible for one of the most common sexually transmitted infections in North America.

Clitoral hood: Prepuce over the superior surface of the clitoris.

Clitoris: Female erectile organ located where the labia minora meet anteriorly.

Closed fracture: Bone fracture not accompanied by a break in the skin. Also called simple fracture.

Colposcope: A lighted instrument with magnification lenses used to enhance visualization of the anogenital structures.

Columnar epithelium: Epithelial cell that is tall and cylindrical, appearing rectangular shaped.

Compound fracture: Bone fracture accompanied by a break in the skin. Also called open fracture.

Consensual sex: Sexual activity that occurs when the individuals involved willingly agree to participate in the activity and are legally able to give permission.

Consensual sex injury: Pertaining to a wound that occurs when engaging in consensual sex. Usually refers to an anogenital wound.

Contusion: A wound that occurs when blunt force ruptures a blood vessel resulting in leakage of blood into the tissue. Also known as a bruise.

Corpus cavernosum: Either of two columns of spongy erectile tissue in the shaft of the penis.

Corpus spongiosum: A column of spongy erectile tissue surrounding the urethra in the penis.

Cowper glands: Glands in the urethral sphincter at the base of the penis that contribute a small amount of fluid to semen. Also known as bulbourethral glands.

Crescentic hymen: Hymen resembling the shape of a segment of a ring.

Cribiform hymen: Hymen with multiple irregular-size openings.

Crust: Collection of dried serum or body fluid.

Cut: Wound caused by dragging a sharp object along tissue. Also known as an incised wound.

Cystocele: Herniation or protrusion of the urinary bladder through the wall of the vagina.

Decomposition: The process by which organic substance breaks down into simpler forms of matter after death. The chemical process involves two stages: autolysis and putrefaction.

Defensive injury: Wound that occurs during the act of defending oneself.

Dentate line: Sawtooth line that divides the proximal and distal anal canal. Also known as pectinate line.

Dentition: The arrangement of teeth in the oral cavity.

Dermis: Layer of skin below the epidermis composed of connective tissue, elastic tissue, nerves, blood vessels, hair follicles, and glands.

Diagrammatic documentation: Documentation using drawings on diagrams or body maps.

Digital camera: A camera that records images via an electronic image sensor.

Digital penetration: Penetration of the anogenitalia by one or more fingers.

Drag mark: Oval-shaped bruise or abrasion on the skin overlying the spinous processes.

Ecchymosis: Hemorrhagic spot or patch caused by extravasation of blood into the tissue. Caused by bleeding of a hematological nature, not trauma.

Ejaculation: Ejection of semen from the male urethra.

Emergency contraception: Medication taken after unprotected sexual intercourse to prevent pregnancy from occuring.

Epidermal inclusion cyst: Benign cyst caused by the implantation of epidermis into the dermis or by an obstructed or malformed hair follicle.

Epidermis: Outermost layer of skin.

Epididymis: Pair of tightly coiled male tubes that carry sperm to the vas deferens from the seminiferous tubules.

Erosion: Superficial loss of epidermis that is moist, without bleeding.

Erythema: Redness of the skin or mucous membrane as a result of dilation of capillaries.

Erythrocyte: Red blood cell.

Estrogen: Hormone responsible for the development of female secondary sex characteristics. Also contributes to the regulation of the menstrual cycle, maintenance of pregnancy, and preparation of mammary glands for lactation.

Evidence-based practice: Provision of healthcare and interventions based on valid, scientific evidence.

Excoriation: Superficial linear abrasions resulting from intense itching or chaffing.

External anal sphincter: Voluntary muscle that forms a broad band on each side of the inferior two thirds of the anal canal that is responsible for keeping the anal canal closed.

External genitalia: External reproductive organs consisting of penis, scrotum, and perineum for males and mons pubis, labia majora, labia minora, clitoris, hymen, and perineum for females.

Fallopian tubes: Pair of tubes that serve as the passage through which ovum is carried from the ovary to the uterus.

Fellatio: Oral sex performed on a male. Consists of stimulating the penis using the mouth.

Fimbriated hymen: Hymen with scalloped projections along the rim.

Finger-pad mark: Bruise caused by pressure of the finger pad or tip during grabbing, holding, pressing, or squeezing.

Fluorescence: Emission of light by a substance that has absorbed light of a different wavelength. In forensics, alternative light sources with ultraviolet light are used to fluoresce substances.

Foley catheter technique: Examination technique that uses an air-filled Foley catheter balloon inserted into the vagina to assist with visualization of an estrogenized hymen.

Folliculitis: Inflammation of the hair follicle.

Fordyce spots: Enlarged sebaceous glands visible through the epithelium of the labia minora.

Foreign object penetration: Pertaining to penetration of the anogenitals by an object.

Forensic examiner: A medical provider who provides medical-forensic healthcare to patients.

Forensic pathologist: A physician specialized in forensic pathology.

Forensic sample: Specimen of body fluid, hair, debris, or other matter used for criminal or civil legal purposes.

Foreskin: Retractable fold of skin that covers the glans penis or clitoris. Also known as prepuce.

Fossa navicularis: Concave depressed area located inferior to the hymen at the posterior union of the labia minora.

Fracture: Injury to bone in which the continuity of the bone is broken.

Frenulum: A fold of tissue that restrains the motion of a mobile organ.

Genital herpes: Viral infection of the genitals caused by the herpes simplex virus.

Genital warts: Viral infection of the genitals caused by the human papillomavirus.

Gingiva: Tissue overlying the alveolar bone that covers the unerupted teeth and encircles the neck of the erupted teeth.

Glans: Erectile tissue at the end of the penis and clitoris.

Grip mark: Bruise pattern that reflects the grip impression left by a hand.

Gunshot wound: Wound caused by the discharge of a gun.

Hard palate: Bony portion of the roof of the mouth.

Health Insurance Portability and Accountability Act (HIPAA): Federal privacy act endorsed by congress in 1996 that provides regulations for the use and disclosure of an individual's health information.

Hemoglobin: Iron-containing protein in the red blood cell that is responsible for oxygen transport.

Hidradenitis suppurativa: Chronic disease caused by hair follicle occlusion that results in obstruction and inflammation of the apocrine glands.

Human immunodeficiency virus (HIV): A type of retrovirus that contains RNA that produces its own DNA inside infected cells. Results in acquired immune deficiency syndrome (AIDS). Transmitted through contact with an infected person's body fluid.

Human sexual response: Refers to the male and female physiological response to sexual arousal.

Hymen: Thin membrane that surrounds or partially covers the vaginal introitus.

Hypervascularity: Increased concentration of blood vessels.

Imperforate hymen: Refers to hymenal tissue that completely covers the vaginal introitus.

Implied consent: Granting of permission for health-care without a formal agreement between the patient and healthcare provider. Usually inferred by the person's actions or inaction and the circumstances of a particular situation.

Incidence: Number of new cases of disease or occurrence in a particular period of time.

Incised wound: Wound caused by dragging a sharp object along tissue. Also known as a cut.

Informed consent: Granting of permission from a patient for the healthcare provider to perform a test, procedure, or provide care after being informed of the relevant facts, risks, and benefits. Informed consent requires the patient to have legal and cognitive ability to grant permission.

Internal anal sphincter: Involuntary smooth muscle surrounding the superior two thirds of the anal canal that is contracted to prevent leakage of fluid and flatus.

International Association of Forensic Nurses (IAFN): International membership organization of forensic nurses who provide leadership in forensic nursing practice.

Keratinocyte: Epidermal cell that synthesizes keratin.

Labia majora: Large lateral folds or lips of the female external genitalia.

Labia minora: Small medial folds or lips of the female external genitalia.

Laceration: Wound caused by tearing, ripping, crushing, overstretching, or shearing of tissue.

Langerhans cell: Dendritic cell of the epidermis that processes microbial antigens.

Lentigo simplex: Benign macule or patch caused by excess melanin production on the labia majora or labia minora.

Lichen sclerosis: Chronic inflammatory disease that results in epithelial thinning, dermal changes, and inflammation.

Lichenification: Area of thickened, leathery skin often caused by chronic irritation from continuous rubbing or scratching.

Lividity: Red to purple coloration in dependent areas of the body due to postmortem accumulation of blood secondary to gravity. Also known as livor mortis.

Livor mortis: Red to purple coloration in dependent areas of the body due to postmortem accumulation of blood secondary to gravity. Also known as lividity.

Longitudinal ridge: Ridge of vaginal tissue that extends the length of the anterior and posterior vaginal walls. Also known as vaginal column.

Macrophage: Phagocytic cell in the immune system.

Macule: Flat area of discoloration on the skin that is less than 1 cm in diameter.

Maggot: Larva of a fly.

Medical-forensic examination: Physical examination of a person by a healthcare provider for medical and forensic purposes.

Melanocyte: Cell in the skin that produces melanin pigment.

Melanosis: Increased pigmentation caused by excess melanin production.

Molluscum contagiosum: Viral infection caused by the molluscum contagiosum virus, a type of pox virus. Predominantly seen on the genitalia, buttocks, abdomen, and thighs.

Mons pubis: Pad of adipose tissue that overlies the symphysis pubis in a female. Also known as mons veneris.

Mucous cyst: Benign cyst caused by obstruction of the vestibular glands.

Mummification: Drying of body tissue after death causing a parchment-like appearance.

Myosin: A protein found in muscle tissue that assists in contraction and relaxation.

Nabothian cyst: Cyst on the cervix caused by occlusion of a mucous gland.

Narrative documentation: Documentation using words and partial or full sentences. Usually refers to documentation of a patient's medical history and physical examination.

Neisseria gonorrhoeae: Gram-negative, diplococcal bacteria responsible for the sexually transmitted infection gonorrhea.

Nevi: Benign skin tumors smaller than 10 mm in diameter.

Nodule: Elevated solid lesion larger than 1 cm in diameter that extends into the dermis.

Nongenital injury: Wound occurring to a body part other than the anogenitals.

Nonconsensual sex: Sexual activity that occurs without a person's consent. Also known as rape or sexual assault.

Nonconsensual sex injury: Pertaining to a wound that occurs during nonconsensual sex. Usually refers to an anogenital wound.

Open fracture: Bone fracture accompanied by a break in the skin. Also called compound fracture.

Oral cavity: Cavity of the mouth.

Oropharynx: One of the three anatomic divisions of the pharynx. Extends from behind the uvula to the level of the hyoid bone and contains the tonsils.

Ovary: Female gonad that produces ova.

Pain scale: Scale that healthcare providers use to measure a patient's pain intensity.

Papule: Superficial, elevated solid lesion less than 1 cm in diameter.

Patch: Flat area of discoloration larger than 1 cm in diameter.

Patterned injury: Wound that possesses characteristics and features indicative of the object or surface that produced it.

Pearly penile papule: Small papule that occurs in rows around the edge of the corona of the glans penis.

Pectinate line: Sawtooth line that divides the proximal and distal anal canal. Also known as dentate line.

Penile shaft: Body of the penis. Composed of the corpora cavernosa and corpus spongiosum.

Penis: Male reproductive organ that forms part of the external genitalia. Serves as a passage for urine and semen.

Perianal: Pertaining to the area around the anus.

Perineum: Area of the body situated dorsal to the pubic arch and arcuate ligaments, ventral to the tip of the coccyx, and lateral to the inferior rami of the pubis and the ischium and sacrotuberous ligaments. Generally referred to as the area between the scrotum and anus in males, and the vulva and anus in females.

Periurethra: Pertaining to around the urethral meatus.

Petechiae: Red, non-elevated bruising that is less than 3 mm in diameter and results from rupture of capillaries.

Photographic documentation: Documentation using pictures taken by camera to record information.

Physical evidence: Objects that can establish that a crime has been committed or provide a link between a crime and the victim or assailant.

Physiologic hyperpigmentation: Natural occurring areas of increased pigmentation generally located on the labia minora and perineum.

Plan B: A type of emergency contraceptive medication taken after unprotected sex to prevent pregnancy.

Plaque: Superficial, elevated solid lesion larger than 1 cm in diameter.

Posterior fourchette: Bridge of tissue formed by the union of the labia minora posteriorly. Also referred to as posterior commissure.

Postinflammatory hyperpigmentation: Increased pigmentation that occurs at the healed site of a trauma or inflammatory condition.

Postmenopausal: Refers to the time after menopause. Applied to women who have not experienced menstrual bleeding for a minimum of twelve months.

Prepuce: Retractable fold of skin that covers the glans penis or clitoris.

Prevalence: Number of all new and old cases of disease or occurrence in a particular period of time.

Primary lesion: Lesion that develops on the skin as a result of a disease process.

Prostate gland: Exocrine gland in men that surrounds the urethra just below the bladder and secretes an alkaline fluid that constitutes approximately 30% of the volume of semen.

Psychological: Refers to behavior and mental processes.

Puberty: Process of physical changes that occur during adolescence enabling the capability of reproduction.

Pustule: An elevated collection of turbid fluid less than 1 cm in diameter.

Putrefaction: Stage of decomposition due to bacteria and fermentation spreading throughout the body.

Race: Refers to a group of genetically related people who share certain physical characteristics.

Rectocele: Herniation or protrustion of the rectum into the vagina.

Rectum: Portion of the large intestine, approximately 12 cm long, just proximal to the anal canal.

Rigidity: A temporary stiffening of the muscles caused by the loss of adenosine triphosphate regeneration and an increase in lactic acid in the muscles after death. Also known as rigor mortis.

Rigor mortis: A temporary stiffening of the muscles caused by the loss of adenosine triphosphate regeneration and an increase in lactic acid in the muscles after death. Also known as rigidity.

Scale: Excess dead epidermal cell that is produced by abnormal keratinization and shedding.

Scar: Permanent fibrotic change in the skin that occurs when normal tissue is replaced with connective tissue.

Scrotum: Pouchlike sac that contains the testes. Part of the male reproductive organs.

Sebaceous glands: Oil-producing glands in the skin.

Secondary lesion: Lesion that evolves from a primary lesion due to the evolution of the lesion, passage of time, scratching, or infection.

Seminiferous tubule: Long coiled tube in the testes where spermatozoa are produced.

Septate hymen: Hymen with one or more bands of tissue that cross the vaginal introitus.

Sex-related homicide: Homicide with evidence of sexual behavior by the assailant before, during, or after the homicide occurs.

Sexual assault evidence collection kit: A kit containing materials for collecting and preserving forensic evidence from the bodies of the victim and assailant after sexual assault.

Sexual assault nurse examiner (SANE): Registered nurse who specializes in providing healthcare to patients reporting a sexual assault.

Sexual assault response team (SART): Multiple agencies that work together to respond to reported sexual assaults within a community. Usually composed of representatives from healthcare, victim advocacy, and law enforcement.

Sexually transmitted infection: Communicable disease transmitted through sexual contact.

Sharp force trauma: Wound caused by a pointed or edged weapon.

Simple fracture: Bone fracture not accompanied by a break in the skin. Also called closed fracture.

Skene glands: Glands that drain into the urethra. Located just within the urethral opening.

Skene gland cyst: Cyst caused by the obstruction of the Skene gland ducts.

Skin slippage: Refers to skin slipping off the body during decomposition after death.

Slap mark: Wound pattern that reflects the outline of the palm and fingers caused by the force of an open hand hitting skin.

Soft palate: Soft tissue suspended from the posterior border of the hard palate responsible for closing the nasal cavity during swallowing.

Speculum: Instrument used to separate the walls of a cavity. Vaginal specula are metal or plastic and shaped similar to a duck beak.

Spermatozoa: Mature male gamete. Also known as sperm.

Squamous epithelium: Epithelial cells that are a flat, platelike shape.

Stab wound: Wound that occurs when a sharp, pointed instrument penetrates the skin and underlying tissue.

Strangulation: Applying external pressure to the neck causing interruption of oxygen exchange to the brain by impeding blood flow or respiration.

Sudoriferous glands: Sweat producing glands.

Suicide: Intentional taking of one's own life.

Symphysis pubis: Cartilaginous joint between the anterior surfaces of the right and left pubic bones.

Syphilis: Sexually transmitted infection caused by *Treponema pallidum*, a spirochete bacteria.

Tanner Stage: A measurement for physical development of secondary sex characteristics. Also known as Tanner scale.

Testes: Male gonads responsible for the production of sperm and testosterone.

Testosterone: Naturally occuring androgenic hormone responsible for the growth and development of male reproductive organs, secondary sex characteristics, spermatozoa, and body growth.

Toluidine blue dye: Nuclear stain commonly used to enhance visualization of anogenital injury. Staining depends on the presence of nucleated cells at the exposed surface. Positive staining can occur with trauma, cancer, inflammation, and other conditions that expose nucleated cells.

Tonsil: Mass of lymphoid tissue on each side of oropharynx that protects against bacteria. There are three types: palatine, pharyngeal, and lingual.

Transverse folds: Transverse ridges in the vagina that allow for vaginal wall expansion and stretching. Also known as vaginal rugae.

Traumatic alopecia: Loss of scalp hair or baldness as a result of forceful pulling of the hair.

Trichomoniasis: Sexually transmitted infection caused by the protozoan *Trichomonas vaginalis*.

Ulcer: Craterlike area of skin that has complete loss of epidermis and at least partial loss of dermis.

Urethra: Small tubular structure that drains urine from the bladder.

Urethral caruncle: Benign outgrowth of distal urethral mucosa.

Urethral prolapse: Protrusion of urethral mucosa through the meatus.

Uterus: Hollow, muscular, internal female organ that is the site of menstruation, implantation, and development of the fetus.

Uvula: Cone-shaped process hanging from the soft palate that helps prevent food and liquid from entering the nasal cavity.

Vagina: Distensible, tube-shaped, fibromuscular canal that extends from the vestibule to the uterine cervix.

Vaginal column: Ridge of vaginal tissue that extends the length of the anterior and posterior vaginal walls. Also known as longitudinal ridge.

Vaginal introitus: Entrance to the vagina.

Vaginal rugae: Transverse ridges in the vagina that allow for vaginal wall expansion and stretching. Also known as transverse folds.

Vas deferens: Duct that conducts spermatozoa from the epididymis to the ejaculatory duct.

Venous pooling: Venous congestion resulting in bluish to red discoloration and perianal swelling.

Vesicle: An elevated collection of clear, serous fluid less than 1 cm in diameter.

Vestibular papillae: Soft, filliform, tubular structures found on the inner labia minora.

Vestibule: Area that serves as an entrance to a passageway. The vestibule of the female external genitalia is bordered by the clitoris, medial aspects of the labia minora, and the posterior fourchette.

Vulva: Refers to the female external genitalia.

Wheal: Superficial, transitory, edematous plaque caused by infiltration of the dermis with fluid.

INDEX

Note: Page numbers followed by f, t, and b refer to figures, tables, and boxes.